Mentoring in General Practice

Mentoring in General Practice

Rosslynne Freeman BA MSc

Visiting Fellow
Royal College of General Practitioners
and
Educational Adviser (General Practice)
Thames Department of Postgraduate General Practice
London University
Guildford
Surrey
UK

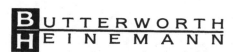

OXFORD   BOSTON   JOHANNESBURG   MELBOURNE   NEW DELHI   SINGAPORE

Butterworth-Heinemann
Linacre House, Jordan Hill, Oxford OX2 8DP
225 Wildwood Avenue, Woburn, MA 01801-2041
A division of Reed Educational and Professional Publishing Ltd

 A member of the Reed Elsevier plc group

First published 1998

British Library Cataloguing in Publication Data
A catalogue record for this book is available from the British Library

Library of Congress Cataloguing in Publication Data
A catalogue record for this book is available from the Library of Congress

ISBN 0 7506 3940 7

Typeset by BC Typesetting, Bristol BS31 1NZ
Printed and bound in Great Britain by Biddles Ltd, Guildford and King's Lynn

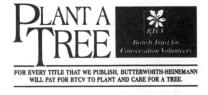

FOR EVERY TITLE THAT WE PUBLISH, BUTTERWORTH-HEINEMANN
WILL PAY FOR BTCV TO PLANT AND CARE FOR A TREE.

In memory of my husband Brian, whose wise counsel and intelligent insights are embodied in these pages, and whose constant and loving support brought the book to completion.

Contents

About the author

Rosslynne Freeman is the Educational Adviser in General Practice for South Thames (West) Department of Postgraduate General Practice Education, and International Education Adviser to the Royal College of General Practitioners. With a background in psychology and higher education, she worked for a number of years combining a university appointment with educational work in general practice, before taking up her present appointment. In addition to her work in promoting mentoring as a tool for professional development in general practice, which has won national and international acclaim, she undertakes to develop the educational skills and knowledge of both general practice and hospital teachers. Her interest in teaching and learning across cultures is maintained by working alongside colleagues from general practice on teaching programmes both at home and abroad.

Foreword

The idea of mentoring is certainly not new and as this book makes clear mentoring goes back to ancient Greek mythology with the example in Homer's *Odyssey* where Mentor is the faithful companion. Rosslynne Freeman reminds her readers that there are many famous mentors in history of world-class importance, including Freud and Jung. The idea of a mentor has, since the early 1970s, been built into the idea of the general practitioner trainer.

Nevertheless, the idea of mentoring does not come immediately to mind amongst those who have participated in a conventional medical education, particularly those reared on the formal lecture and large ward rounds. This book shows, however, that mentoring has taken its place as one of a number of important developments in adult education and one which draws roots from many disciplines. Rosslynne Freeman interprets it mainly through the social science perspective of educational psychology with liberal quotations from related disciplines.

Mentoring should logically appeal more to general practitioners than to most other groups of doctors, since no other discipline is based so centrally on the one-to-one consultation with a variety of people and deals with such a wide variety of problems.

This book describes mentoring, both in theory and practice, and focuses on using reflective discussion as a means of encouraging professional development. Rosslynne Freeman considers the theory, which she bases on Kolb cycle, and discusses the knowledge, attitudes and skills needed by those who are to be mentors and the implications for both parties. Throughout she focuses on the human and personal aspects of mentoring rather than the alternative emphasis on management and on organisational theory.

The impact of mentoring may also be particularly great in general practice. Branthwaite *et al.*[1] showed that many general practitioners have low self-image. There is certainly a traditional problem of isolation and general practitioners provide about 15 consultations per week on average more than in almost any other country in the Western world. High volume through-put associated with isolation is a recipe for loss of reflective capacity. Mentoring is one mechanism whereby this can be reintroduced into practice. It is also a particularly comfortable model since it enables the skills of experience to be shared, and indeed this book makes the point that retired general practitioners can function as mentors thereby maintaining a considerable resource within the profession.

Mentoring will not suit everybody, nor should it be made compulsory, but for those who value reflective discussion and for those who are prepared to learn in a variety of ways, the extension of mentoring offers substantial hope and encouragement as a powerful learning method particularly suited to general medical practice.

Twenty-five years ago general practice adopted the interactive small group as a then new and powerful educational method which proved exciting and liberating for a variety of general practitioners. Now it seems likely that mentoring, although a very different method, may produce equally exciting results.

Rosslynne Freeman can be congratulated on a thoughtful and reflective book which does much to set mentoring in its place on the educational scene.

Denis Pereira Gray
General Practitioner, Exeter
Professor of General Practice, University of Exeter
President, Royal College of General Practitioners

1 Branthwaite A., Ross A., Henshaw A. *et al.* (1988) *Continuing Education for General Practitioners. Occasional Paper 38*. Royal College of General Practitioners, London.

Preface

Rivers, ravines and bridges – developing mentoring in general practice

The intention of this book is to tell a story. Like all good stories, it is told on different levels, and has different layers of meaning. It ends happily, with a beginning – those questions still to be answered, tasks yet to be undertaken, another story to be told.

At an academic level, it is a commentary on the development of mentoring in general practice, used as a strategy for professional development. It is told through the medium of a 3-year research project which established a continuing mentor scheme in South West Thames.

The first part of the book reflects the sequence of the four phases of that work: identification, formulation, implementation, and review. Chapter 1 addresses the first phase, in which an attempt was made to identify more clearly the forces operating at the time when 'mentor' and 'mentoring' became popular words in a profession struggling to come to terms with a new order, and which formed the context of the study. The second chapter reviews significant literature from other professions experienced in the art of mentoring, comparing these other definitions of the role and function of a mentor with that envisaged by general practice.

Chapter 3 is in four parts. The first part focuses on formulation, and tells of the design of a holistic model of mentoring. It was devised after a period of careful exploration and discussion with general practitioners to identify what sort of mentoring would most effectively meet the perceived needs of practitioners. It shows how the design of the model was shaped and influenced by the issues described in the two earlier chapters, whilst the second part describes a strategy designed to aid the establishment of an effective mentoring relationship. In the third part the experience of introducing the holistic model of mentoring to general practitioners interested in acting as mentors is described. The fourth and final part of the chapter considers requisite skills in mentoring.

Chapter 4 – the implementation phase – offers a picture of holistic mentoring being used in practice, with some emerging strengths and weaknesses discussed. Obstacles encountered in its introduction are described, and the reviews and amendments made to keep it on course are outlined.

The story of mentoring is developed in the following two chapters, and moved to a deeper level. In Chapter 5, an account of the structure and experience of using reflective practice to further the professional development of the mentors is given, and this is followed in Chapter 6 by written contributions from two mentors, who tell of their experience of taking on the role, and summaries from four recipients of mentoring, the mentees.

No attempt has been made to edit these contributions and bring them into line with the overall writing style of the book, for as the central characters in this story, it is important that they speak for themselves.

The outcomes of the mentor's intervention are more formally addressed in Chapter 7, where the action-research framework of the mentor project is introduced. The outcomes of the internal evaluation of the project are summarized, before two independent researchers describe how they went about an external evaluation of the application of the holistic mentor model.

Chapter 8 introduces the theme of diversification. In the first part of the chapter, important aspects of culture and gender in the mentoring process are discussed, and illustrated by examples from practice. A further illustration of diversity is provided in the second part of this chapter, where a different form of peer support is described.

Towards the end of the story some practical guidance is offered for those who are encouraged to begin their own journey of exploration. Chapter 9 is intended as a 'do-it-yourself' step by step instruction for mentor project instigators. It does not guarantee success, but like all other chapters in this book, is intended to play the part of a metaphorical mentor – acting as guide, who has undertaken a journey, and is prepared to share their experience with those who are just starting out.

As there can be no ending to this tale, the final chapter reviews the moral of the story, and reflects on some of the issues that are raised in its telling, including those (as yet) unanswered questions, which accompany the developmental journey of mentoring as the profession moves from one state of being to another.

For the author, it would of course be satisfying to join the honourable ranks of those who can confidently assert that their work has contributed significantly towards increasing the knowledge base of their particular subject; but experience shows that it is frequently the readers who pay the price for such nobility, as they plod wearily through the dense forest of references and complexities. With this in mind, I have tried to keep the story in the foreground although as the story is not fictitious, it is underpinned by referenced evidence. For those readers who enjoy seeking morals in stories, the text overleaf offers the entire story of mentoring in general practice, upon which to reflect.

The first phase of work, which sought contextual themes to explain the proliferation of mentoring in medicine, was seen from the outset as crucially related to the final outcome of the research project. The context into which new initiatives are born shifts and changes over time, sometimes rapidly; understanding and identifying some of the surrounding factors that usher into being a new idea makes forecasting necessary adaptations to that idea easier, and more accurate. As the context changes the initiative needs to be adapted, so that it continues to be 'needs-responsive'. This includes considering the point at which the initiative is no longer necessary – if the context of general practice changes as rapidly as it has in the last 5 years, will we still need mentors? Why did we feel we needed them in the first place?

'When Allah the Merciful and Compassionate first created this world, the earth was smooth and even as a finely engraved plate. That displeased the Devil who envied man this gift of God. And while the earth was still just as it had come from God's hands, damp and soft as unbaked clay, he stole up, and scratched the face of God's earth with his nails as much and as deeply as he could.

Therefore, deep rivers and ravines were formed which divided one district from another and kept men apart, preventing them from travelling on that earth that God had given them for their food and their support. And Allah felt pity when he saw what the Accursed One had done, but was not able to return to the task which the Devil had spoiled with his nails, so he sent his angels to help men and make things easier for them.

When the angels saw how unfortunate men could not pass those abysses and ravines to finish the work they had to do, but tormented themselves, and looked in vain, and shouted from one side to the other, they spread their wings above those places and men were able to cross.

So men learned from the angels of God how to build bridges, and therefore, after fountains, the greatest blessing is to build a bridge, and the greatest sin to interfere with it, for every bridge, from a tree trunk crossing a mountain stream to this great erection of Mehmed Pasha has its guardian angel who cares for it, and maintains it as long as God has ordained that it should stand.

So it is, by God's will.'

(Traditional Ottoman tale translated from the Serbo-Croat by L.F. Edwards. In *The Bridge Over the Drina* (ed. Ivo Andric). Harvill Press, London (paperback edition 1994)).

Acknowledgements

My first debt is to the mentors, from whom I have learnt much about myself, the art of mentoring, and the profession of general practice. This book is a testament to their pioneering achievement, and any failure to convey the accuracy and worth of their work is mine, and not theirs.

Dr Robert Clarke instigated the idea of writing a book, and by his own enthusiasm for new ideas, persuaded me that it was manageable, and enjoyable. On balance, he was right, and I am grateful to him for his advice on getting started.

The loyal support of the Dean of Postgraduate General Practice Education, Dr Rimon Hornung, is acknowledged with much appreciation, both in his continuing commitment to the development of mentoring in South Thames (West), and his individual attention in reading the early draft of the manuscript.

Laura Lawrence has on many occasions prevented my descent into author-dementia by her sensible advice, and constant encouragement. Finally, my thanks go to the contributors for the additional dimension which their work provides.

1

Context of mentoring in general practice: Mismanagement of organizational change

'there is nothing more difficult to execute nor more dubious of success, nor more dangerous to administer, than to introduce a new order of things; for he who introduces it has all those who profit from the old order as his enemies, and he has only lukewarm allies in all those who might profit from the new'

(Machiavelli[1])

> This chapter considers the context into which mentoring was born, and sets the background scene to the mentoring story, using frameworks of crisis and change as vehicles for discussion. The detrimental effects of imposed change are considered and some of the symptoms of dis-ease presented by the profession in response to a changing climate discussed. The potential of general practice education as a helping or hindering force in the adaptation to change leads to the emergence of the mentor, and closes with a contemplation of their future role.

Concepts of change and crisis

The continuing background to the development of mentoring in general practice is the crisis of organizational change. Change does not take place in isolation from other social, economic and political factors, and from these factors come helping and hindering forces, undercurrents which predict either a stormy passage for the change process, or fair winds to blow it on its course. The impact of these forces is influenced by the nature of the change, whether it be foreseen and carefully planned, or sudden and ill-informed. The latter introduces the element of crisis, which, like change, has within it the seeds of its own resolution, although at the time they appear remarkably dormant.

Side by side with the threat of change, sits opportunity – the Taoist belief of opposing forces existing within the whole. The crisis of change threatens continuity, and throws us into unstable and uncertain states. Given certain conditions, the experience of the crisis of change, though traumatic and dishevelling, can result in new insights which add positively to a way of life, so that crisis is not simply survived, but learnt from.

Murray-Parkes' seminal work on bereavement[2] showed that for some individuals the terrible crisis of loss brought some gains which enhanced their life. These positive outcomes depend on the availability of helping forces – that they exist, can be sought out and strengthened, and can be made easily available to an organization or an individual – so that the disruption of change is supported by a helping framework.

The manner in which the new order of general practice was introduced was in itself a hindering force, creating as it did more enemies than luke-warm allies. Perhaps because of this, there was a heightened need to strengthen existing helping forces, and create new ones. The seeds of creativity in the profession survived the turmoil, growing into a number of initiatives which had as their objective the development of the ability of individual practitioners to come to terms with change, and the new demands being placed upon them.

The experience of 'living through' change reminds us that it is not a single event, but a process, a journey from one state of being to another. The familiar world recedes and with it known objects, familiar practices are lost. The new world is at first unfamiliar, and contains unknown and unforeseen demands; it requires exploration, and a process of adaptation to new circumstances. Some individuals, faced with such uncertainty, doubt their ability to find their way around, or whether they have sufficient emotional and physical energy to sustain the adaptation. This leads them to resist change, and fight to maintain the status quo, sometimes with justification – 'if it ain't broke, don't fix it'.

The change journey moves through different phases of reactions, towards an outcome that may, or may not, be positive and rewarding. Whether a positive outcome is achieved is influenced by those factors in operation when the change process began, and in this respect, change models are strongly related to crisis models, and the stages model of grief and mourning. Fink *et al.*'s model[3] provides a useful introductory framework of individual change (Table 1.1).

Table 1.1 Introductory framework of individual change

Phases involved	Perception	Emotion	Behaviour
Shock	Reality of threat is accepted	Helplessness, fear, panic, loss	Withdraws, blaming
Defensive retreat	Dismissive of proposed change, continues to work with existing structures, clings to familiar	Appears calmly indifferent, unconcerned, easily angered	Celebrates the past, behaves as if everything remains unchanged, delights in evidence of chaos
Acceptance	Confronts reality, gives up existing structures, devalues own ability to work with new	Depression, grief, resentment, resignation to change accompanied by bitterness	Do I fit anywhere? Reluctant joining
Adaptation and change	Perceptual shift Integration of new experience (or maladaptation to change)	Increasing enthusiasm Recognition of positive experiences Gradual increase in satisfaction	It might work this way . . . We could try . . . Not as bad as I feared

Adapted from Fink *et al.*[3]

In the late eighties and early nineties, family doctors spoke of their realization of threat to the existing situation, and their fear that the changes to their working structures were unrealistic and unworkable. There was a general sense of shock, and feelings of helplessness about the ability to influence the outcome of impending changes to working structures which were seen as unrealistic and undesirable.

At both an individual and organizational level, Caplan's crisis model[4] adds further features to the model of the change process. Two of these are closely related to the outcome of the crisis, and influence the organization's ability to adapt to changed circumstances, either negatively – in which case the organizational crisis is simply survived – or positively, meaning that the change is made to work to the organization's advantage. They are, firstly, those factors present in the life of an organization or individual at the point of entry into change and, secondly, the availability of support at a critical phase of the journey, referred to in Figure 1.1 as the 'window of opportunity'.

When individuals and organizations are emotionally robust and in good health at the point of entry into a change crisis, with an intact and functioning support network, the prognosis for their eventual adaptation to it, and the possibility of a positive outcome, is heightened. Conversely, if at the start of the change process they are fatigued, or emotionally depleted, struggling with economic problems or the threat of redundancy, these factors act as negative stressors, making for a poorer prognosis for the outcome of the process, in the same way that patients already in a lowered state at the onset of an illness will take longer to recover.

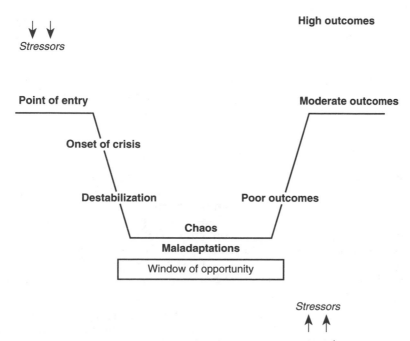

Figure 1.1 Caplan's crisis model. (Adapted and developed from Caplan[4])

Crisis is seen as a downward journey, a slide towards a low point. In the descent, we find that previous coping strategies fail, furthering a sense of chaos. We hit the bottom, where all known strategies have been tried, and all attempts to get out of the crisis have failed. But, in this nadir of the journey is the 'window of opportunity' where, faced with the realization that all efforts to reverse the slide have failed, we are less defensive, less resistant to the intervention of others, and more open to the possibility of learning new strategies. Critical to this stage is the second relevant feature, that of the ***presence*** or ***absence*** of helping forces which lift us out of the mire, upwards, and outwards towards a newly integrated life.

In the absence of available support comes a heightened risk of maladaptations to the crisis. At their lowest point, people seek relief from their helplessness and panic through inappropriate means, for example the abuse of drugs or alcohol. Occasionally suicide is seen as the only way out. A further maladaptation comes in taking on inappropriate roles, frequently that of patient, for this provides an honourable retreat from a turbulent world, providing shelter in an illness. These maladaptations are critical, for they mean that individuals never totally regain their former position. Their adaptation to the crisis of change leaves them in some way diminished – emotionally, or physically, or simply worse off economically and socially than when they went into it – leading to the worst outcome. Others will simply survive the crisis, coming out at the same level of entry – a moderate outcome, whilst others will learn and develop from their supported experience, making gains which mean they exit from the process at a higher level than where they entered.

There are, of course, more positive aspects to crisis – the dormant seeds of resolution. One is the element of relief. When the crisis breaks, energy absorbed in previous imaginings is re-directed into active confrontation of the event, and emotionally this is preferable to living in a state of anxious anticipation. Crisis catapults individuals and organizations into a new-found state of determination to overcome – there are few things more likely to unify a workforce than a common enemy, and no group as powerful as one where enemies and lukewarm allies unite to devise strategies by which to survive the threat.

At the point of entry into organizational change which surrounded the introduction of the New Contract were, then, two pre-existing factors likely to make the adaptation process more difficult:

- Firstly change was imposed. Change did not originate from within the profession, as a natural evolution arising from the experience of practice; furthermore, and as commented upon earlier, it was imposed from outside, by powerful yet distant authority without a proper process of professional participation and consultation.
- Secondly, it was imposed upon an already stressed profession, amidst growing concerns about raised mortality in general practice from suicide and alcohol abuse, the detrimental effects of out-of-hours work, and falling recruitment.

The beginning of the mentor's tale is set, it seems, amidst a turbulent world in which a vengeful Devil is intent on spoiling that which was pleasing, creating the sort of havoc which keeps men and women from travelling around for their food and support, choosing instead to stay safely at home with the doors closed on the outside world – an unlikely scenario into which to introduce mentors. To become a helping force, rather than another hindrance, mentors would need to appear to their colleagues as being relevant to the time and place on the journey of change, and to achieve this, it was important to clearly understand how these concepts of change and crisis were experienced by doctors, and manifested themselves in their daily working life.

Detrimental effects of imposed change: professional issues

The detrimental effects of imposed change are well rehearsed, clearly and relevantly summarized by Scott and Marinker:[5]

'when change is perceived as having been willed by others rather than occasioned by need there is a sense of arbitrariness. The new contract . . . is an obvious example. It was the sense that activities were willed as a matter of policy, politically decided and enforced by a monopolistic employer or commissioner, that caused the sense of helplessness and hopelessness' (p. 1548).

The lack of appropriate and comprehensive consultation for the imposed change meant that it lacked credible evidence from the profession, who felt no sense of ownership of the measures inherent in it, or identification with its aims. As this is a prerequisite for the successful implementation of change,[6] it is not surprising that many practitioners voiced their strong opposition to it. Equally important, it influenced at the outset the likely outcome of the objective. Adaptation to change is strongly influenced by whether the workforce has been involved in the setting of objectives, planning and implementation of the change process. When change is not well managed, both individuals and organizations are likely to spend longer in the defensive phase, making the process of change traumatic, and protracted, and diminishing the likelihood of its objectives being met.

The second factor was the organizational state of health of the profession as it went into the change process – the point of entry. Margaret Thatcher's radical reform of the National Health Service (which began in 1988) led ultimately to fundholding, through the introduction of the internal market in medicine, with GPs and health authorities as purchasers, and hospitals as providers. This created a professional climate which emphasized competition, not co-operation, setting doctor against doctor. Fundholding created a divide between those practitioners who saw it as a rightful opportunity to empower general practice, and those who thought the price of such empowerment struck at the very roots of the unique doctor–patient relationship. When a new contract was imposed upon general practitioners – in effect implementing change through a coercive power relationship – it brought further competition for patients, through the introduction of target payments and performance related pay. Additional stress factors came from the vast administrative structure evolved to support a contracting process, which demanded practitioner time and involvement. A further dispiriting factor was the evident drop in recruitment to general practice, as medical students, sighting the combined minefield of the New Contract and the NHS reforms, opted to stay in hospitals or switch to a less demanding profession. Taking the New Contract in 1990 as a professional crisis, it would be reasonable to assume that at the point of entry into Caplan's crisis model, the organizational health of the profession was far from robust.

Fink *et al.*[7] follow their model of individual responses to change with a second which details the phases of organizational reaction to change (Table 1.2). This shows how an organization's leadership responds to the imposition of change. The risk of fragmentation means that an organization is divided into different factions, which fight amongst themselves – another bonus for the envious and displeased Devil. For example, the role of the Royal College of General Practitioners as a major player in organizational change was never clear – criticized by some as being passive in the face of change, it was said by others to have conspired to bring about negative change, and upbraided by others for not representing the profession's views strongly enough. Another view, based on Fink's organizational model of response to change, would be one of a leadership paralysed by the swift implementation of the imposed change, and still attempting to manage its own response to threat.

The background to this specific organizational change were the wider, continuing changes occurring in society. The recession affected most people's lives in some form, and redundancy in particular, previously seen as the province of an unfortunate few, became common; people's confident expectation of a stable working life, and one which ended in a retirement cushioned by a state pension, was ended. The pattern of continuous work, with its surrounding framework of a mortgage and a desired lifestyle, was replaced with short-term contracts of work. Tenure in professional posts became a thing of the past, and portfolio careers were introduced as the passports to a new, and exciting future – provided that you had transferable skills.

Table 1.2 Organizational reaction to change

Phases involved	Interpersonal relations	Leadership and decision making	Problem solving	Organization structure
Shock	Dysfunctioning and/or fragmented	Paralysed and/or controlling	Reactive and/or absent	Chaotic
Defensive retreat	Protective and cohesive	Shifts between uncertain/ autocratic	Procedural Cautious	Traditional Defensive
Acceptance	Supportive Cathartic	Democratic Participative	Incorporates change: creative	Experimenting
Adaptation	Interdependent	Task-centred	Exhaustive and integrative	Evolving and developing

Adapted from Fink *et al.*[7]

Perhaps to balance the increasing sense of powerlessness engendered in the population by such insecurity and change, the Government of the day introduced measures aimed, it seemed, at empowering the individual, but in fact signalling a move towards a culture of administrative accountability. Public service departments were required to set out and publish their objectives; league tables and other measures of their achievements were introduced. Clients and patients became 'customers' and 'consumers' who could hold the service to account for the quantity and quality of their care, and any perceived failure to provide it. The Patient's Charter, setting out the rights of patients, but saying less about their responsibilities towards their doctor, serves as an illustration. In a prime example of mismanaging change, the Accursed One (taking the form of the Government) had scratched deeply into the damp clay of general practice, changing its relatively smooth face forever. Existing ravines were widened by this act, and others were created. In either case, the detritus of mismanaged change added to the disarray.

Detrimental effects of mismanaged change: issues of professional and personal stress

In this period of upheaval and change, peering in from outside, members of other professions looked enviously at doctors, held in the eye of the storm, guaranteed work for life, with fair and adequate financial recompense, and then viewed reports of increasing levels of stress in the medical profession with some cynicism. Those on the inside knew the paradox – that a society reeling from structural change finds its way first and foremost to the surgery:

'you ask about stress factors in our lives? I will tell you the biggest – out there are hundreds of people who have lost their jobs, have had their houses repossessed, are terrified that a day off sick will cost them their job, that if they don't meet impossible targets that they spend 16 hours a day chasing they will be replaced with someone who can – it makes them feel sick, ill, frightened. And they bring all this to me and put it on my desk, every day, and they want me to do something, to make it better, to reassure them that it will be OK. And it isn't OK. I can do nothing to help them – how can I change society?'[8]

Social factors influence the consultation, and the nature of the general practitioner's workload. The turbulence of major societal change meant many members of the population sought their GP's help in alleviating the continuing symptoms of change-related illness – anxiety states, reactive depression, and stress. At times of social change, the patient's unrealistic expectations of a doctor's heroic ability to change situations for the better may be heightened, which in turn heightens the feelings of helplessness experienced by the doctors, as they face the insurmountable problems laid before them, and feel the distress of their patient.

An additional factor for the already-harassed doctor was the continuing decline in the levels of satisfaction with the doctor–patient relationship.[9] As patients became more informed and more critical, general practitioners were no longer held in such personal high regard, nor the profession with as much respect and prestige as in the past.[10] The rapid development of information technology over the past 15 years, and a campaigning media, has led to an increasing availability of knowledge once held to be the domain of the profession. Patients are more informed about their condition and available treatment, more able to enter into discussion about ways of responding to their illness, and consequently more critical of their doctor's performance. The mystique of any profession is eroded when the knowledge gap between the professional and the consumer diminishes; the professional becomes more ordinary, and less distant. This change in status is further evidenced by the growing number of formal complaints against doctors.

Perhaps perversely, these factors served only to increase rather than to diminish the patient's expectation of what could be done for them, and the publication of the Patient's Charter was an additional provocative factor. It further empowered the consumer, but fuelled unrealistic expectations of what the National Health Service could provide for them.

Existing stressors at the 'point of entry'

Into a professional group already working at the coalface of societal change, and into the existing ravines of patient demand, practitioner stress and deteriorating status, was imposed a New Contract of work, the effects of which on the professional population are well documented.

Following the implementation of the Contract, and against a background of widening research identifying stress factors, the British Medical Association's 1992 published report[11] focused growing concern on the hitherto largely hidden problem of stress in the medical profession. The report, it seemed, gave permission for stress to be brought openly into the arena for discussion, encouraging the funding of further research activities, and enabling the Royal College of General Practitioners to appoint its own 'Stress Fellows' to consolidate a stress database, and educate practitioners in stress reduction and coping strategies.

Emerging from the copious literature on job-related stress in general practice, seven identified stress factors for general practitioners emerge, which pre-dated the imposed New Contract:

Demands of the job – the inconsistent nature of the work which defeats attempts to organize and plan a manageable working day
The unrealistic expectation of patients, and their lack of appreciation
Interference with family life – the invasion of family life, and lack of privacy when living in the same community as patients
Being on call
Constant interruptions at work and at home
Patient complaints
Practice administration.

As the Contract became reality, further study sought to identify the responses of general practitioners in terms of their level of job satisfaction, and the stress which they experienced in coming to terms with the new working requirements. This research showed further related stress factors piling into existing ones:

Increased paperwork and bureaucracy
Further increase in patient demand
Increased accountability for efficiency
Loss of control over work pattern and direction
Litigation.

All of these contributed significantly to a reduction in job satisfaction, and increased stress, as two seminal studies, comparing levels of stress amongst practitioners before and after the introduction of the New Contract[12] clearly show.

How did this stress manifest itself in the ordinary working life of practitioners? Much has been written about occupational stress in relation to medicine, and it is not the purpose of this chapter to repeat it, but instead to isolate those stress factors which impinged upon practitioners' attempts to come to terms with imposed change. Moreover, these factors were seen as hindering forces as the profession moved towards the third phase in our model of change – acknowledgement, acceptance, and the beginnings of adaptation. If not recognized, they would act as negative stressors, likely to divert the energy of practitioners away from adaptation to change, and were therefore important considerations in the development of a mentoring model.

Conflict with partners

The contract brought into family medicine a different element – a business element, with managerial roles, and mission statements, greater emphasis on competence and accountability, finance-related targets, and competition with others. For many practitioners, then and now, the new component sat uneasily with the traditional model of continuing care for an entire family group 'from cradle to grave', and risked eroding the fundamental core of general practice – the consistent relationship with a known and trusted 'family' doctor, lovingly portrayed by the media through such popular classics as *Dr Finlay's Casebook*. Other doctors embraced wholeheartedly the opportunity of fundholding, to control the purchase of care for their patients, compete in the healthcare market place, and streamline their practice with an eye to maximizing profits as a successful small business. And it left many doctors somewhere in the middle, pondering whether it were possible to maintain the strengths of traditional caring for patients, whilst at the same time reaping the benefit of a more 'value for money' organized practice, able to exert greater influence on the shape of a primary care led future health service.

Such tensions challenged professional values, and served to widen one organizational ravine already in place, but little reported – conflict between partners in a group practice. Such conflict can range from transient but recurring differences which deplete the energy source of practitioners, to full blown hate and festering divisions which make professional life a misery. In an early paper which reviewed the literature on occupational sources of stress, Cooper and Marshall[13] suggest that good relationships between members of a work group are central to good health, and that mistrust of the persons one worked with led to inadequate communication, psychological strain, low job satisfaction, and a feeling of threat to one's wellbeing.

The New Contract obliged doctors to consider their inner beliefs about what was important and central to the practice of family medicine, imposing as it did a demand for services which many practitioners did not perceive as clinically appropriate, or necessary. It demanded the take-up of managerial roles, about which many doctors were uncertain and unprepared for, lacking appropriate training. It gave voice to the discord between individual beliefs, professional values, and the demands of a new era, heard in passing remarks – 'this is not what I trained for', and 'I didn't come into general practice to be doing this [usually referring to a managerial task] – I came into practice to see patients', and in so doing, it made some of the inherent divisions within a practice overt, and more stressful.

A common form of expression of 'difference' is in consulting styles – between those doctors perceived as 'patient-centred', who prefer to hold longer consultations with patients and whose surgeries take longer and see less people, and those 'doctor-centred' practitioners with shorter consultation rates, who get through surgeries faster. In a practice with an undeclared, or uncertain collective belief, there is more room for value judgements to be made on different styles of working, creating division. Whilst practical strategies for rectifying the outcome of different practice styles exist,[14] this is best achieved when the values that underpin the difference have been aired, and their implication understood. As Howie *et al.* cite, all is possible within the context of good interpersonal relationships within the practice, seen as a firm support when they are good, and a major source of stress when problematic.

Personal autonomy

The nails of the Accursed One also scratched deeply into the sense of personal autonomy and control hitherto enjoyed by doctors, and deemed to be the significant determinants of professional, as opposed to non-professional life.[15] After 1990, there was a heightened sense of accountability, with an accompanying decrease in autonomy:

'I am no longer in charge of my professional life – but dancing to someone else's tune – and a very discordant tune at that.'[16]

Karasek's model of job strain details a positive correlation between the high job demand of general practice, and high 'job decision latitude'.[17] A highly demanding job was less stressful, and more enjoyable, when there was equally high freedom of latitude to act autonomously in decision making and planning, and this was supported in Cooper and Sutherland's later study,[18] where the authors commented that high demands on doctors' time, heavy workloads, and responsibility for others became intolerable burdens when personal autonomy was removed.

In proposing an alternative to the New Contract, Morrell[19] comments that the contract determined standards of performance which were concerned almost entirely with preventive care, some of questionable benefit, and which seemed to ignore the right of patients to accept or reject care.

Overall, the contract was imbued with the belief that 'good care', as defined, would attract more patients to the good doctor, who would receive financial reward through the capitation system – a belief which ignored the crucial aspect of primary care, which Morrell described as being

'the time doctors can devote to listening and identifying their patients' problems . . . providing counselling, advice, health education, and appropriate management' (p. 1005).

This is an activity closely aligned to 'the art' of general practice, the indefinable, yet unique aspect of patient care borne out of the continuing relationship with the patient, which goes beyond the mere treatment of disease. In describing four ways in which general practice is different from other specialities, McWhinney[20] describes the first as being the way in which the discipline defines itself in terms of relationships, especially doctor–patient relationships. The new order further diminished professional autonomy by denying the unique and different nature of general practice, predicting the content and process of the consultation, organizing treatment around clinics and protocols, thus reducing the autonomous practice of medicine

'to a form of art which is no more creative or responsive than painting by numbers' (p. 1549).[21]

Role conflict

This experienced loss of professional autonomy appears closely related to another identified stressor – role conflict.

Role conflict exists when an individual in a particular work role is torn by conflicting job demands, by doing things he or she does not want to do, and does not perceive as being part of the job specification. Relevant to the story of mentoring are three related components of role conflict: organizational, professional and personal.

Overall changes in the demands and expectation of the role of a family doctor in the 1990s were embodied in government edicts for organizational change, communicated to the profession by a powerful but distant group (the Government). Organizational role conflict is significantly heightened when an individual, or a professional group, are

'caught between two groups of people who demand different kinds of behaviour or expect that the job should entail different functions . . . the greater the power or authority of the people "sending" the conflicting role messages, the more job dissatisfaction is produced' (p. 16).[22]

This led many doctors to examine their new, different professional role in relation to their partners in the practice group. Some doctors experienced personal feelings of a misfit between their individual self and their working environment, made manifest by covert and overt messages from partners. Thirdly, role conflict was expressed in the interface between personal, family life and professional life. Increasing demand took its toll on personal life, where doctors felt torn between the reasonable expectations of their life partners and families for quality time together, and resentful of the increased demands which made them unable to provide it.

Conventionally (and medicine is conventional), women are viewed as the primary victims of stress arising from conflicting roles, as they balance work with family life, torn between their career and mothering their children. As male and female roles become less stereotyped, driven by a society where the traditional breadwinning role of the male is eroded through redundancy and/or the greater earning power of their partner, the desire of some men to take a more equal share in the physical care and emotional nurture of their children becomes more overt. Myerson's work[23] suggested that, whilst women GPs are stressed by the lack of flexibility in general practice, the competing demands of home and work, and the reductionist effect of part-time working on their pension, male GPs also find the integration of work and family life problematic.

Research from the sociological perspective suggests that male doctors may not always be aware of it. Bates,[24] discussing the implications for the doctor–patient relationship when doctors cannot cope with their own stress, interviewed the spouses of 84 general practitioners asking them to respond to the question 'is he emotionally drained when he comes home?' Four out of five general practitioner wives said yes, he was, frequently – and cited examples by which they assessed this depletion, particularly noting the length of time it took for their doctor-partner to unwind after work, and their generally withdrawn state. When asked the same question, only one out of four of their doctor–partners regarded themselves as 'frequently' emotionally drained, seeing themselves rather as 'physically tired'. Those doctors who were prepared to accept that they experienced some emotional stress said that

'after supporting other people all day, something must rub off on the supporter' (p. 33).

For these doctors, (and many outside the study) home was a sanctuary from work, and this meant that they did not want to come home to be greeted with family problems – a fact recognized by spouses, who described their endeavours to shield their partners from their own problems and concerns. The potential for further stress resulting from this unnatural state of affairs is obvious, and is described in further studies.[25]

Responses to a questionnaire used in the pilot study, which preceded the mentoring work described in this book, indicate that some practitioners attempt to separate work from personal life by not discussing work matters with their spouse, although the majority used their personal partners as their main support. Those who did so commented in ways which suggested that they were mindful of the deleterious effect of overloading their personal relationship with the more negative concerns of work. This was particularly relevant when there was conflict with their partners in practice, particularly where a social relationship existed which involved their spouses.

The emotional exhaustion referred to above (frequently unrecognized by the individual who gradually adopts a cynical, negative attitude towards their work, depersonalizing patients in order to maintain emotional distance which will defend them against overwhelming stress), is an important concomitant of burnout. Burnout, a graphic if emotive term, describes a state of psychological and physical depletion, insidious in onset, characterized by withdrawal into cynicism, feelings of exhaustion and apathy, accompanied by somatic symptoms, depression, and excessive use of alcohol.[26] In a study which set out to examine the extent of burnout in general practice[27] it was seen that young practitioners were more at risk than older, established colleagues, and that the availability of sufficient time out, to counterbalance the demands of time at work, reduced the threat.

One pragmatic solution to stress then, is to reduce workload and take time out – organizational stress would be reduced if more practitioners became part-time. Those practitioners who have been able to do this might well confirm that they fare better – but the pressures on practitioners from patients and partners alike were to *increase* their workload, to play their part in meeting new targets, and meeting increased demand. For those stressed practitioners in the middle of their careers, the economic prospect of working less was prohibitive – and added a further stressor:

'I feel trapped – I can see no way out of a profession that, ironically, I slogged for years to get into . . . for what else could I do? Medical training doesn't equip you to do much more than be a doctor . . . and where else would I earn a salary to keep the kids at school and the mortgage paid?'[28]

The lack of any overt career structure in general practice means the individual practitioner has to be very self-directed in finding the means of their continuing stimulus and professional development. This self-motivation has to exist alongside opportunities to put ideas into action, when neither exist, the feeling of being trapped in one job for life is emphasized.

Continuing education as a helping and hindering force

Part of the new order clearly signalled the increased personal account-ability of the practitioner for their continuing competence, manifested in the educational buzz words of the time, as doctors were urged to become 'lifelong learners', planning and undertaking continuing educa-tion which was appropriate to their identified learning need, relevant to the task in hand, and benefiting patients through improved care. This call for increased accountability sat uneasily with decreased autonomy and, in an attempt to redress the balance, brought into focus ownership of educational change. Educators in general practice talked increasingly of 'learner-centred learning' and began to find ways of offering 'self-directed' learning programmes designed to put the doctor back in charge of his or her educational journey. If practitioners had not yet got owner-ship of change, they could at least have ownership of their professional development.

It is perhaps worth moving aside for a moment or two to revisit the his-tory of educational independence in general practice, to see again why it continues to be a strong, helping force, strong enough to weather most political interventions and setbacks. From 1850, medical education was exclusively in the control of hospital based specialists, and this remained so until the 1960s, despite the 1882 working party of the British Medical Association's Metropolitan Counties branch noting that 'no inconsiderable number of recently qualified medical men have any idea of the real duties of general practitioners until they are actually engaged in practice'. This was compounded by the implicit, and explicit, attitude of medical schools which favoured medicine practised in hospitals, by hospital doctors, preferably working in a teaching hospital. General practice was an occupation one turned to when the higher echelons of 'real' medicine were closed to you, and the prevailing attitude towards family doctors as 'failed' consultants continued the low status of general practice within the medical profession. Although the 1911 National Insurance Act initiated the framework for current general practice, and was incorporated into the National Health Service in 1948, it was the hospital based doctors who dominated the planning and were appointed to the prestigious posts. Family doctors were offered lower financial rewards, which only emphasized and continued their relatively low status. Recruitment to general practice was so low that hospital doctors could walk in and find an immediate position, without further training. Further erosion to generalist medicine came from the vast leaps in knowledge made in the 1950s which narrowed the focus on specialism, so that, correspondingly, patients seen in hospital beds became less and less representative of general medicine.

Against this background, with morale in general practice at a low ebb, came the Cohen Report[29] making authoritative suggestions for 3 years of specific training for general practice. And a further upturn followed in 1952, when, in the face of strong opposition from sections of the medical profession, the Royal College of General Practitioners was formed and gave some sense of collective identity to general practitioners. When the Doctor's Charter of 1965 heralded improved pay and working conditions, there was a platform from which to campaign for general practice as a specialism of its own within the medical profession. The vehicle to express independence was vocational training – and the newly formed Royal College seized the opportunity with vigour. The sleeping giant was awakening to overcome its long standing educational deprivation,[30] and, in so doing, further assert its independence.

This shift away from the confines of medicine into the broader perspectives of postgraduate professional education can be clearly observed in the literature emerging from the 1970s, which shows that the models of training for general practice which evolved were embedded in the basic principles of adult education, and even today remain in stark contrast to the constriction of hospital-based learning. Moving teaching towards the perspective of the patient as a 'whole' person, not simply a diseased body, gave validity to knowledge residing in other disciplines contributing to understanding of human behaviour – psychology, sociology, philosophy. This wider panorama took in a further dimension – the relationship between the doctor and his or her patient, and the human interaction of the consultation. The relationship between teaching and learning was acknowledged, so that effective teaching moved well beyond imparting necessary skills to include the management of attitudinal change in the learner, and an ability to motivate their desire to change. Continuing education in general practice became firmly rooted in the soil of education, rather than science, a trail blazing move which carried not only educational intent, but a declaration of the independence of general practice.

Perhaps because of this historic struggle to become an independent discipline, the reins of general practice education have remained firmly in the hands of general practitioner educators. 'In house' educational events are most usually constructed and delivered by educators from within the profession, most of whom retain their commitment to practice, combining an educational role with their clinical work. This has the sound advantage of maintaining the credibility of the teacher, who, with their feet also planted in the everyday experience of general practice, cannot be set aside by their student's as 'not understanding' professional issues, and places the educator in an excellent position to gather first-hand the emerging educational needs of his or her peers. The downside has been to muddle educational agendas, and to regard education as the panacea for all professional ills, with a tendency to disregard the equally unique knowledge of other disciplines. There is still an element of surprise when general practice opens its doors to outsiders and finds that they import relevant and useful new perspectives, nicely summed up by Neighbour:[31]

'I wish medicine could teach other disciplines half as much as they can teach it'.

Education in general practice then is rooted in the concept of lifelong learning – more fashionable now in a society where disrupted employment patterns demand wider application of knowledge, acquired not in one intense and final block in early adult life, but dispersed throughout a lifetime, tied more closely to the workplace, and continuing from early to late adulthood. This already-familiar knowledge, and years of experience of not only peer learning in the workplace but also peer review of such learning, was a strong positive force in setting about meeting the demand for increased accountability through evidenced, continual professional learning. But this helping force had to surmount the hindering force of the struggle to adapt to the organizational change, a struggle which left many practitioners more concerned to survive the demands of the clinical week than review their future learning needs. In Maslow's hierarchy of need, the bottom of the pyramid is concerned with meeting and consolidating basic needs of shelter and security – self-esteem comes much higher up, the icing on the cake as it were. The provision of funding in the early 1990s which offered educational initiatives for inner-city general practitioners in London showed clearly that, however good the educational programmes on offer, first and foremost came the provision of locum cover which freed the doctor to leave his or her practice without loss of income, or reprisal from overworked partners having to shoulder yet more patient care – basic needs first.

From the perspective of a professional educator, and crucial to the development of any new initiative, was the essential factor of freedom to learn. GP educators are a resourceful lot, in themselves a helping force, but it was clear that many of their imaginative innovations would founder simply because prospective participants were busy coming to terms with increased workloads, surviving their practice conflicts, too embittered to raise their heads above the parapet, or were simply exhausted. They were not, as Carl Rogers described[32]

'free to learn . . . for man is not free, but controlled by factors beyond the self' (p. 46).

Unless new educational innovations, albeit designed to strengthen helping forces, could acknowledge the blocks to that essential freedom to learn, and address the fall out from imposed change, they would be seen as yet another demand upon a demoralized workforce. They would be undertaken half-heartedly to earn the postgraduate education allowance and offer proof of attendance, rather than an opportunity of exploring, working with, and managing the threats posed by the required change.

Summary

The context of the development of mentoring in general practice was of a profession caught in the movement between the destabilizing low point of crisis, marshalling its resources to make the necessary adaptation to an imposed new order. The mismanagement of organizational change accentuated existing negative forces within the organization, and introduced further obstructions to the positive progress of the change process – described in this chapter as hindering forces.

Surrounding the point of entry into change were two critical factors. Job-related stress factors meant that many practitioners were faced with change when they felt personally depleted, demoralized, and undervalued. In such a climate, the ready availability of support structures became more necessary, but less likely, as the profession was already under siege, struggling to survive the ordinary demands of daily practice. The strongest helping force identified was the profession's long history of producing effective educational measures to support practitioner development, but this was a double edged sword when accountability for continuing education was seen as a yet further demand on time and energy.

At the nadir of crisis is the window of opportunity, presenting at the lowest point of the crisis, sitting steadfastly alongside the threat of change. One of the greatest threats of the new order lay in its sharpening of competitiveness between general practice colleagues, lessening co-operation, and diminishing even further the sense of collegiality recalled wistfully by many established practitioners, but seen as belonging to the past. The lack of this camaraderie meant that for some practitioners ravines became an abyss, leaving them tormented, looking in vain for a way to cross the divide, yet not shouting too loudly, for whoever heard their shouts might perceive them as failing, and be tempted to take advantage of their struggle.

This particular threat carried within it the seeds of its own resolution. The Accursed One, in creating ravines, made it impossible not to notice that they existed. With stress firmly in the public domain, and on the profession's agenda, came permission to speak more openly of the deepest river keeping men and women apart in general practice, that of the defensive nature of medicine, an organizational climate, in which the doctor has to appear at all times to be all-coping and infallible – the mask of relaxed brilliance.[33] The majority of doctors wish to fulfil their own, and their patients' expectations of them as being invincible, and medical training has taught most doctors to avoid sharing feelings of anxiety, or uncertainty, for fear of being labelled as weak, not up to the rigours of clinical medicine.

In this window of opportunity, the historical defensiveness of medicine was questioned, and defences were lowered sufficiently to contemplate a means by which the profession could develop 'in house' support structures, and begin to look after its own. The rise in the use of the word 'mentor' coincided with this time of threat and opportunity.

From their Homeric inception, mentors have been seen as those (traditionally older and wiser) who support another (usually younger and inexperienced) to make a safe transition from one state of being to another, helping to overcome obstacles in a journey towards a new way of being. Although in general practice the word was often used to describe activities very different from those commonly understood elsewhere as 'mentoring', it did appear that the mentor's proposed function consistently included an element of support.

Were mentors envisaged as helping forces who would seize the opportunity to lessen the isolation and divisions brought about by change, and move the profession towards regaining sight of its strengths and rewards? Or were they a gentle disciple of the threat of accountability, did the name imply the velvet glove on the iron fist of re-certification, appraisal, and re-accreditation? Were they simply the by product of educational fashion, intrinsic to the development of the self-directed learning movement – or, as in higher education, pawns in the political game to replace academic professional education with competency-based training in the work place?

The obvious answer is 'yes' – to all, in part. But a wider perspective on the role and function of mentors in organizations is gained through reviewing how other professions have deployed mentors – for, contrary to the belief of many, general practice did not invent mentoring. Why did other professions include mentors in their organizational structures? What function were they expected to serve, and how might they have benefited the organization in which they operated?

References

1 Machiavell N. 1961 *The Prince* translated by N. Bull. Penguin Books, Harmondsworth, London
2 Murray-Parkes C. 1972 *Bereavement – Studies of Grief in Adult Life*. Pelican, London
3 Fink S. *et al.* 1971 Organisational crisis and change. *Journal of Applied Behavioural Science*, **7**, 15–41
4 Caplan G. 1969 *An Approach to Community Health*. Social Science Paperbacks, London
5 Scott M.G.B. and Marinker M. 1992 Imposed change in general practice. *British Medical Journal*, **304**, 1548–50
6 Beckhard R. and Harris R.T. 1987 *Organizational Transitions: Managing Complex Change*. Addison-Wesley, Reading MA
7 Ibid
8 Data from field notes, Surviving General Practice workshop, October 1996
9 Cartwright A. and Anderson R. 1981 *General Practice Revisited*. Tavistock Press, London
10 Cooper C.L. and Sutherland V.J. 1992 Job stress, satisfaction, and mental health among general practitioners before and after introduction of the new contract. *British Medical Journal*, **304**, 1545–8
11 *Stress in the Medical Profession* – Supplementary report of the British Medical Association (collective publication). British Medical Association 1992

12 See Cooper C., Rout U. and Faragher B. 1989 Mental Health, job satisfaction and job stress among general practitioners. *British Medical Journal*, **298**, 366–70 and, Sutherland V.J. and Cooper C.L. 1992 *British Medical Journal*, **304**, 1545–8

13 Cooper C.L. and Marshall J. 1976 Occupational sources of stress: a review of the literature relating to coronary heart disease and mental ill health *Journal of Occupational Psychology*, **49**, 11–28

14 Howie J., Porter M. and Heaney D. 1993 General practitioners, work and stress. Chapter 4 in *Stress Management in General Practice*, Royal College of General Practitioners Occasional Paper No. 61. Published by The Royal College of General Practitioners, London, August 1993

15 See for example Bucher R. and Strauss A. 1961 Professions in process. *American Journal of Sociology*, **66**, 325–34

16 Comment from respondent in the pilot study, South Thames (West) Mentor Project, April 1994

17 Karasek R.A. 1979 Job demands, job decision latitude, and mental strain: implications for job re-design *Administrative Science Quarterly*, **24**, 285–308

18 Ibid

19 Morrell D. 1989 The new general practitioner contract: is there an alternative? *British Medical Journal*, **298**, 1005–7

20 McWhinney I.R. 1996 The importance of being different. *British Journal of General Practice*, July, 433–6

21 Scott M. and Marinker M. ibid

22 Cooper and Marshall, ibid 1976

23 Myerson S. 1997 Seven Women GPs perceptions of their stresses and the impact of these on their private and professional lives. *Journal of Management in Medicine*, **11**(1), 1997

24 Bates E. 1982 Doctors and their spouses speak: stress in medical practice. *Sociology of Health and Illness*, **4**(1)

25 See, for example, Pereira J. and Gray J. 1982 The doctor's family: some problems and solutions. *Journal of Royal College of General Practice*, **32**, 75–9

26 See Freudenberger H.J. 1974 Staff burn out. *Journal of Social Issues*, **30**, 159–65

27 Kirwan M. and Armstrong D. 1995 Investigation of burnout in a sample of British general practitioners. *British Journal of General Practice*, **45**, 259–60

28 Comment of delegate in educational workshop on surviving stress in general practice, October 1996

29 Cohen Committee, 1950 *General Practice and the Training of the General Practitioner*. British Medical Association

30 Pereira-Gray D. 1979 *A System of Training for General Practice*. Occasional Paper, Royal College of General Practitioners, London

31 Neighbour R. 1992 *The Inner Apprentice*. Kluwer Academic Publishers, London

32 Rogers C. 1983 *Freedom to Learn for the 80s*. Charles Merrill Publishing, Columbus OH

33 Coombs R.H., Perell P. and Ruckh J.M. 1990 Primary prevention of emotional impairment among medical trainees *American Medicine*, **65**, 576–81

2
Reviewing the literature: Mentoring in other professions

'In much wisdom is much grief – he who increases knowledge increases sorrow'
(Ecclesiastics 9.11)

In order to show more clearly how the classic role of a mentor has been adapted over time, to produce the phenomenon of modern mentoring, this chapter begins with the original source story of Mentor. As medicine is founded on apprenticeship, we then consider what, if any, relationship exists between apprenticeship and mentoring, before moving on to explore how mentors are seen and used elsewhere. To achieve this, we review some of the relevant literature from four disciplines with a long tradition in mentor-type relationships – nursing, higher education, business and the helping professions. How mentors are defined within those different settings, what role they undertake, and what benefits they are seen to bring to their organization are summarized, before considering how this review further informed the design and implementation of a holistic model of mentoring.

Part 1: Mentors and apprentices: Historical dimensions and medical traditions

The original Mentor appears in Homer's Odyssey.[1] Odysseus (Ulysses), King of Ithaca, faced with 20 years of fighting the Trojan wars, sought the help of his wise and faithful companion Mentor in putting his house in order prior to his long absence. Mentor was charged with overseeing the upbringing of his young son Telemachus, guiding him from childhood to adulthood, preparing him for eventual reunion with his father, and his own future role as king. Mentor was responsible for the boy's education, instilling appropriate values that would shape his future decision making. Years passed and, with his father showing no signs of returning, Telemachus set out to search for him. Mentor accompanied him on his journey, supporting and guiding him when critical choices had to be made. Athene, the goddess of wisdom, intermittently assumed Mentor's form, so that the gift of insight became associated as 'god-given'. At the end of the journey, Telemachus had matured both inwardly in spirit, and outwardly, in being able to manage life events and function independently.

This story, and the fairy stories of other cultures that came later, embody the concept of transition. Young people are faced with a series of obstacles that have to be overcome in order to achieve the desired goal – be it a sleeping princess, or reunion with long lost parents. In the journey towards achievement, various personalities intervene, offering practical insight into ways of overcoming the current obstacle that lies in the path, guiding the individual through transitional stages. In the Greek myth, Mentor was a consistent companion, the transitional figure in Telemachus's journey from childhood to manhood.

Within this Homeric tradition, mentors become synonymous with fatherly protection, guidance, and wise counsel. Virgil, in Dante's *Divine Comedy* takes on a similar guiding role, urging his charge on, protecting him from threat, clearing the way forward, and offering a supportive and trusting relationship within which his charge can develop. Shakespeare frequently cast servants in the role of protector and counsellor to their masters, seeing them as equals in the game of life, even if apparently sub-servient. In his play *As You Like It*, Adam, faithful servant and protector of Oliver, and a conscientious, upright veteran of family disputes, guides Oliver to safety in the Forest of Arden before quietly disappearing from the story.

Alongside fatherly care, Mentor also gave Telemachus some coaching which prepared him for a future responsible role. The Hippocratic Oath* also embodies the idea of a quasi-family situation in which a pupil must regard his teacher and his teacher's relatives as if they were his own, implying the same paternalistic quality found in Homeric mentors, and being bound by this bond to keep the secrets of medicine within this extended professional family. But, as the teaching of medicine expanded, those who had money could pay to gain entry into the family circle.

Writing about medicine in the Greek world between 800 and 50 BC, Sutton[2] describes the increasing professionalization of medical practice, with workshops for medical healers, public medical appointments, lectures in the local gymnasium – and medical taxes. This rapid emergence of medicine as a profession encouraged one prominent Egyptian to appren-tice his son to a 'medical clysterer', confident that he would gain

'an income for life' (p. 37).

In a book which offers for comparison ways in which the healers in the three great scholarly traditions of medicine (Galenic, Chinese and Ayurvedic) claimed to know something about health and healing, Sivin[3] tells the story of a medical student as a disciple, guided in his learning of the art of medicine by an experienced 'knower', whose own personal and professional status is an important aspect of the student–master relationship.

So far so good then, for it appears that medicine was founded on the master–disciple association, which embodied some traditional Homeric values. But this story introduces another aspect which lies at the core of mentorship – the notion of a process of initiation, which, only if success-fully accomplished by the student, allows him access to his master, to begin the process of acquiring knowledge.

In this process of initiation into a culture lies the second core aspect of mentoring – transition, the passing from one stage to another in which some kind of transformation is made. Fairy tales are good examples of

* A translation of the Hippocratic Oath is included at the end of this chapter.

transition. The prince sets out to claim his princess, but finds all sorts of obstacles in his search – he must first chop down thickets of thorns and kill the dragon blocking the entrance to his dream. When he claims her, he claims also his manhood, and can then live happily ever afterwards. Children have to find ways of surviving the wicked witch in a forest of uncertainties and threat, before arriving safely into a better world, prompted in finding their way by the unexpected appearances of the good fairy.

A vivid example of a transitional journey comes from Buddhism, where the noviciate arrives at the temple with his bundle of belongings, and is kept outside, deliberately spurned and rejected by community. This is the first hurdle in his journey, in which his motivation and inner strength are assessed. If he overcomes this first hurdle, he is allowed entry into the community, and thereby access to knowledge.

If this sounds extraordinarily familiar to doctors who have survived the rigours of medical training, there is more to come, for, once inside, our noviciate shares with the student-disciples of Greek medicine similar experiences on their learning journey. Both students are now given access to written texts to read, memorize, and reflect on, but obstacles are placed in their way which make their course of study more onerous. There are accompanying demanding physical preparations – they have to undertake rigorous exercise, forego sexual intercourse, abstain from eating meat, meditate, and undertake long periods of fasting. From time to time, the student doctor is examined on his knowledge by the Master, who, like the Zen Buddhist teacher, is fond of asking unanswerable questions, until such time as he, the disciple, is seen to satisfy the requirements of knowledge.

Modern mentoring relationships recognize that having the knowledge is not, in itself, sufficient to pass from one state to another. Induction into a professional culture is only the beginning of a transitional journey. Again, this movement is apparent in the early examples of student–master relationships – both the Buddhist and the doctor already have their master's knowledge, memorized from the written text, but now each has to internalize this knowledge, reflect further, and be guided verbally in its application by his master. He then becomes

'a legitimate successor in the line of scholars who will keep the text in use, protecting it and teaching it to the next suitable person' [my emphasis] (p. 186).

In this way he moves through *possessing* knowledge of health and healing to *passing* the knowledge on – he becomes a master himself, within the context of a tightly closed medical community – the forerunner of today's GP trainer.

The medical groups that existed in ancient Greece furthered the concept of guided tutelage, given within closed groups that appeared even then as elitist. They were the forerunners of the medieval craft guilds, which continued the principle of monitoring and protecting emergent professionalism, through the apprenticeship model.

Apprenticeship is described by Lipsey[4] as a rite of passage which has three stages – apprentice, journeyman, and finally master. The trials and tribulations of the apprentice are compensated for by the privilege of guided learning under the impressive tutelage of an experienced teacher. Learning is not limited to the technical craft itself, but includes introduction to professional customs, history, and attitudes – all features which grow to resemble later descriptions of a mentor's role. Once basic knowledge is accrued, the apprentice becomes a journeyman – taking on some teaching duties of his own, but more in order to learn than to teach, until he presents his masterpiece – a piece of work which gives evidence of his acquired learning. With this, he asks for admission to the Guild – as a fully fledged professional in his own right.

The trainer–registrar relationship in general practice mirrors this route of induction and transition exactly. The registrar has survived the obstacles of initiation – the ward rounds, the absence of obvious teaching through telling, and answered the apparently unanswerable questions of the exams. He or she presents to the GP trainer as a journeyman (or woman) – to be finished off, inducted into the art of using the acquired knowledge in the real world. If the trainer does his or her job well, then the registrar in turn 'teaches . . . the next suitable person'.

GP registrars, like mentees, are hopeful of finding the 'right' trainer or mentor who will be helpful to them in this transition and, as we shall see later, finding a doctor with experience of the craft was deemed to be essential for our earlier apprentices. The status of the trainer – as the 'master', the 'experienced knower' – is considered as important today as it was then. The trainer must be known, and widely acknowledged by peers as a respected member of his or her profession. Whilst respect might be seen in conjunction with seniority, this is not always the case, and provision is made for this in the training regulations, which state that trainers will 'usually, but not always' have been in full partnership for over 5 years.

The Apothecaries Act of 1815 was the first attempt to regulate the practice of medicine, by requiring those who aspired to practise to become apprenticed to an *experienced* apothecary. The following illustration of a medical apprenticeship shows how even then the profession was beset by defining a 'good' trainer. One aspiring doctor, a Thomas Piggott, was apprenticed to John Meredith, a barber-surgeon, who had something of a private practice as well as a post at the Bethlehem Hospital in London. Dissatisfied with the way the apprenticeship was going, Thomas's father brought a suit against Meredith. Evidence was given to the hearing of Thomas's aptitude and diligence under his master's tutelage, whilst his master did not get such a good report:

'he[the master] would often tymes give to . . . Thomas very ill and bad language, calling him rogue, rascall, and fool, and a puppye, and would often times curse him to ye very greate discouragement of . . . Thomas' (p. 228).

Further testimony was given by a porter and 'keeper' at the Bethlehem (which then housed lunatics) that Thomas never neglected his master's business, either at home or at hospital. The court found in favour of Thomas the apprentice, but later on, when he became in essence a 'journeyman' signified by his becoming his master's assistant surgeon, he was told by his master that he would not employ him as such. Thomas left his master, and went home, whereupon his irate parents once again took up his cause, asking the barber-surgeon to take him back, and when he refused, once more took their complaint to court. This time the apprentice fared less well, for evidence of his drinking was given by other apprentices, who told that court that once, when he returned from the madhouse:

'he was very much disguised with drink . . . and once lost his plasterbox and sayd he had left it at the shoppe' (p. 229).

whilst his master was more convincingly reported as ensuring Thomas was well cared for:

'[he did] keep a very good house and to provide and furnish his servants very sufficiently with all necessary accomedcons [sic] of meate, drink, washing and lodging and all others and to treat his apprentices kindly' (p. 229).

The transitional journeys of today's medical apprentices show a remarkable similarity to that of Thomas the apprentice – the rituals of leaving the parental home and establishing a personal and professional identity are still marked by drinking revels, arriving late for lectures, and losing stethoscopes.

The growth of the apprenticeship model in medicine gave to the profession much of its continuing prestige. Apprentices to London surgical staff comprised the single most numerous groups of the eight medical societies active in London between 1795 and 1815. These societies were formed as gentlemen's professional clubs, which essentially upheld the earlier concept of tutelage within a closed, privileged group. They had as their stated aim being 'desirous of improvements in medicine',[5] a laudable objective which presumably, like membership of RCGP and other specialist colleges, serves both to raise standards and create a hierarchy of professional membership. These groups of master-surgeons, focused in the two main London hospitals Guy's and St Bartholomew's, taught younger members and apprentices, disseminated new theories and techniques, built libraries, and promoted professional unity. These eminent men took on the role of nurturing young aspirants to the profession, and their apprentices formed an elite class. As medicine began to teach its art to groups of apprentices in the 'teaching' hospitals, rather than through individual tutelage, the first written accounts describing individual mentoring relationships appear.

A particularly intense relationship between William Osler – a great practitioner and teacher of medicine in the 1800s – and the Canadian physician James Bovell charts the consistent influence of Bovell from Osler's youth, a man who inspired intense devotion in the young Osler, and to whom Osler dedicated his seminal work *Principles and Practice of Medicine* in 1892.[6] Unfortunately, little is told of the nature of their relationship, for the account focuses primarily on the achievements of both men, but the intensity and consistency of the relationship are obvious, with some evidence that Osler sought the advice and support of Bovell throughout his professional life. Interestingly, Barondess[7] (himself a surgeon) writes of a 'paradigmatic' mentoring relationship between Osler and one Harvey Cushing, where Osler acted as a personal and professional adviser to the young Cushing, ushering him into the world of medicine, suggesting that those who receive mentoring are perhaps more willing to offer it to others.

From its Greek inception, mentoring in medicine appears as male dominated, but examples from the early years of nursing tell of mentoring relationships between women,[8] one such being the mentoring relationship between Annie Goodrich – born in 1866 and achieving remarkable successes in her career – and Anne Maxwell. Anne gave to Annie calm reassurance, generosity of time for talking through her ideas, wise counsel, and psychological support, all of which, it is said, cultivated latent qualities in Annie Goodrich, enabling her to become a prominent leader in the field of nursing.

We begin to locate in these accounts a historical basis in medicine of apprentice-type teaching relationships, and some of the desirable qualities of a mentor. From the Homeric tradition the mentor appears a person charged with an almost sacred responsibility, necessitating that they possess honourable qualities. Protection and support are important, giving rise later to the French protégé – someone who is protected. The mentor's personal power and authority to influence – the ability to open doors and ease the path of the mentee – occurs intermittently. Were these original attributes embodied in the later definitions of a mentor?

Some definitions

Defining the task of a mentor in today's workplace is complex business. Whilst mentors are to be found at work in the professions of nursing and teaching, and in many commercial institutions, they do not always have a clear job definition, nor are the qualities desired in a mentor clearly delineated. In the absence of a clear definition, it cannot be assumed that authors writing about mentoring are talking about the same thing, and indeed the more one pursues the literature, the clearer it becomes that there are many different perceptions of the role, purpose and activity of a mentor. Consistency lies in the *lack* of an overall, clear definition of the word 'mentor'. Merriam,[9] somewhat impatient with this state of affairs, says:

'its meaning appears to be defined . . . by a particular setting in which it occurs'

and gathers force for a concluding statement:

'. . . mentoring is not clearly conceptualised, leading to confusion as to what is being measured or offered as an ingredient of success. Mentoring appears to mean one thing to developmental psychologists, another thing to business people, and a third thing to those in academic settings' (p. 169).

Some writers have confined themselves to searching for a definitive definition. Carruthers,[10] in a wide ranging excursion, begins at the beginning with the Homeric model of Mentor as a father figure, and goes on to identify the roles of teacher, role model, approachable counsellor, trusted advisor, a challenger and encourager in the mentor function. He offers that as Athene sometimes assumed the role of mentor, women are not debarred from practising these skills, even if only occasionally.

Dictionary definitions include the word wisdom, a quality certainly required for those mentors aspiring to Carmin's[11] somewhat daunting definition:

'Mentoring is a complex, interactive process occurring between individuals of differing levels of experience and expertise which incorporates interpersonal or psychosocial development, career and/or educational development, and socialisation functions into the relationship. This one-to-one relationship is itself developmental, and proceeds through a series of stages which help to determine both the conditions affecting and the outcomes of the process. To the extent that the parameters of mutuality and compatibility exist in the relationship, the potential outcomes of respect, professionalism, collegiality, and role fulfilment will result. Further, the mentoring process occurs in a dynamic relationship within a given setting.'

Admirable in its lucidity, and sufficiently ambiguous to cover the variety of mentoring relationships being practised.

Most authors understandably define mentoring from both their own core discipline, and the context of the work being described, resulting in core agreements with peripheral differences. Carruthers[12] helpfully disentangles from the plethora of definitions two distinct categories:

1. Those which emphasize the professional development of the protégé only
2. Those which emphasize both the professional and personal development of the protégé.

This distinction is taken further by Philips-Jones[13] who defines mentors as being

'influential people who significantly help you reach major life goals.'

But, when an emotional bond develops, the protégé is deemed to have a 'primary' mentor, whilst 'secondary' mentors are those who have a considerably lighter impact on the protégé with little emotional bonding. This widens the field into considering the existence of transient mentors, who may be helpful to the development of an individual at a particular time, but have no sustained relationship. Thus a number of mentors may emerge spontaneously over a life period, linked to dominant professional and or personal issues of the time, who do not necessarily possess all the classic mentor ingredients.

The importance of a mentor to personal development is central to the work of Levinson *et al.*[14] who base their work on psycho-social and psycho-dynamic theoretical frameworks of developmental psychology. Implicit in their text is Winnicot's[15] concept of 'good enough parenting' – Levinson *et al.* suggest that there are 'good enough' mentors who are less than ideal, but adequate in a practical sense. Their work on the developmental nature of the mentoring relationship, with the central concept of transition, has had a profound influence on the understanding and practice of mentoring, and will be revisited in following chapters.

Similarly Darling,[16] a major commentator in the field, emphasizes the quality of the relationship between mentor and mentee. In discussing its influence on the mentee's life, she differentiates between whether the mentor is a major, or minor one, and deducing that a major mentor is a more profound and valuable influence for the mentee. Her work is returned to in the following discussion on mentoring in the nursing profession.

In summary, Jacobi[17] concludes that there is

'continued lack of clarity about the antecedents, outcomes, characteristics and mediators of mentoring relationships'

but nevertheless goes on to offer no less than fifteen mentoring functions derived from research. These reflect three components of the mentoring relationship:

1. Emotional and psychological support
2. Direction assistance with career and professional development
3. Role modelling.

(p. 510)

At this point in the review, it seems that the gain of wisdom through acquiring knowledge of mentoring definitions brings only the grief of confusion. However, there is a consistent theme of context, which suggests that the style of mentoring is consistently adapted to the needs of the organization in which it takes place. My own analysis of this theme suggests that this adaptation of the mentor's role to the needs of the organization is arrived at by varying the weighting given to the potential components of the role – emotional support, assistance with career development, role modelling, etc. – dependent upon the perceived needs of the organization. The heaviest weighting is the area from which the role and function of the mentor is then derived, and described. To test this understanding further, let us begin an exploration of the declared role and purpose of a mentor in three very different settings: nursing, education, and the business world – in order to identify what (if any) consistent applications appeared which might be then be viewed as 'core characteristics' of a mentoring relationship.

Part 2: Mentoring in nursing

Kramer[18] would appear to have paved the way for the establishing of mentoring in American nursing with her concept of 'reality shock'. Any adaptation to a new culture or role can be seen as a challenge, or a threat. When academic, theoretical learning for a professional role is undertaken in isolation from the reality of practising it in real life, the moment of applying theory to practice brings more trauma, and heightens vulnerability – which can overwhelm the student practitioner, to the extent that they leave the profession. Her work produced the idea of assigning mentors – usually first level nurses – to these students, to act as wise and reliable counsellors who would help the students cope, reducing the high fall out rate. It is exactly for this reason that, 20 years later, there is growing interest in providing mentors to support junior hospital doctors to confront the reality of practice.

Almost all the descriptions of mentoring in nursing refer to American models, with Darling[19] appearing as a consistent commentator. In her extensive work on the characteristics of the mentor, she is adamant that there are three vital ingredients to mentoring *'so vital, in fact, that if one is missing, the mentor relationship becomes minor, or secondary'* (p. 43).

The three vital ingredients described are:

Attraction: Where the mentee is attracted to the mentor by admiration and the desire to emulate

Action: The mentor demonstrates that they have the time/energy and appropriate behaviours to act on the mentee's behalf

Affect: Respect, encouragement and support for the mentee are evident.

These three ingredients are correlated with the mentor taking up the three dominant roles: inspirer (attraction), investor (action) and supporter (affect), roles which were later expanded through her extensive research to include the mentor acting as a role model, supporter, standard-prodder, teacher, career counsellor and challenger.

But Morle[20] argues that the whole concept of mentoring in the nursing profession is inappropriate, making him critical of the cavalier attitude to mentoring schemes:

'in this country (UK) the absences of a clear definition of the role, function, and preparation of the mentor does not seem to have hindered in any way the ready uptake of the idea' (p. 67)

and goes on to speculate that the most compelling force for the uptake of mentoring in the nursing profession owed little to altruistic desire and more to political expediency – the need to comply with an English National Board directive, and questions whether the variety of supportive roles available in nursing constitute the 'mentor' label, as they appear as precarious and inconsistent. It is not difficult to see the parallels in general practice.

The term 'preceptor' would appear to describe a more appropriate role in nursing than mentor, in that it is more closely tied to clinical practice. Echoing this, Chickerella and Lutz[21] define preceptorship as:

'an individualised teaching/learning method in which each student is assigned to a particular preceptor . . . so that she can experience day to day practice with a role model *[my emphasis] and resource immediately available within the clinical setting.'* (p. 17).

Armitage and Burnard[22] compare the role of mentor and preceptor. The mentor role is seen as benign, the mentor stands back and allows the student to develop in autonomous ways, acting as facilitator, or surrogate parent. They see the role of a preceptor as being

'more clinically active and more of a role model than the mentor. The preceptor is more concerned with the teaching and learning aspects of the relationship, whilst the mentor, although concerned with these things, seeks a closer and more personal relationship' (p. 226).

This preceptor concept moves mentoring away from a broader, pastoral relationship with the strong emotional bond implied by Darling, to a more defined focus on learning from a good role model.

In one of the few British research studies Gerrish,[23] using a small qualitative design, focused on aspects of the transition process made by nurses as they begin to work on the ward, and describes the haphazard manner in which nurses learnt their new role. The staff nurses felt inadequately prepared, feeling that their student status during training had shielded them from some of the situations they were now encountering – for example, breaking bad news to relatives of dying or critically ill patients, and coping with bereaved relatives following patient death, seen by all respondents as the most stressful professional encounter. Clinical training had not included training in delegation, negotiation, and decision making, yet, faced with these problems, participants in the study did not always seek guidance from the obvious source – from their first line manager. Three reasons were given – firstly, they did not find their manager approachable, secondly, they doubted her credibility, perceiving her to be out of touch with current practice, and thirdly, they felt that their own credibility as a nurse was viewed in terms of their ability to function independently of support and guidance. This is another aspect which strongly resonates with general practice, when the trainee general practitioner becomes a junior partner in a group practice, and appeared relevant to my own later findings on the experience of mentees.

In their refreshingly straightforward and lucid book, Morton-Cooper and Palmer[24] tell of how confusion over the terminology of support roles has dogged clinical practice in nursing and midwifery, particularly when it comes to preceptors and mentors. Their own understanding of the difference supports that of Morle's[25] view of the preceptor as a role model, whilst mentors are associated with training programmes, and learning support. This confirms that a consistent theme of both preceptor and mentor models is supported learning either assisting:

the *integration* of new learning commensurate with taking up a different role

or

the *application* of theoretical teaching to practice experience.

Is this theme replicated when mentoring in educational settings is explored?

Part 3: Mentoring in the context of higher education

In education, the primary context for mentoring is in teacher-training, where once again the mentor acts to support the theory-into-practice function of professional learning. Wilkin[26] provides an invaluable collection of essays on mentoring in higher education, beginning with an overview of the development of the mentoring role in education.

Prior to the mentoring role being established, teachers on training practice merely received hints and indirect advice from their training supervisor on how to develop teaching skills. In 1987 the Department of Educational Studies at Oxford University introduced an 'internship scheme' where 'interns' (student teachers) on placement were paired with a mentor, an experienced teacher in their subject, under the supervision of a third person, a professional tutor. The philosophy of the scheme came from the belief that whilst the taught component of teaching training in college was valuable and distinctive, teachers in schools were best placed to develop teaching skills in students – a similar philosophy to that which now urges an undergraduate curriculum placed in the community, not the hospital. Government ratification of this scheme confirmed an important shift – away from teachers who supervised students and saw that they put into practice what they had learnt at their training institution – to schools taking direct responsibility for the provision of structured, consistent on-the-job training, carried out by qualified personnel (mentors).

This began the continuing move in education to equalize the power base of training by more closely relating theory to the reality of practice, and honouring the importance and skill of a good 'practice teacher'. From this base, the role of the mentor in education was clearly defined:

1. To arrange, or initiate a number of training tasks with the student
2. To provide confidential and clearly focused discussion of professional experiences
3. From these, to identify the learning needs of a student and construct an appropriate programme to meet them.

This original model of mentoring was defined by the context in which it developed. The absence of any personal relationship, or friendship, between the mentor and student, with no counselling or interpersonal skills demanded, reflected the tradition of an ancient university where such an inclusion would be seen to contaminate the intellectual activity of teaching teachers to teach.

Looking at more contemporary models, Black and Booth[27] provide a more reasoned view for excluding a personal dimension – the need for mentors to actively engage in non-threatening evaluative feedback to the student, as no learning gains were made if the mentoring relationship was oversupportive, collusive, and non-critical. But Hurst and Wilkin[28] set out guidelines for mentors which imply the possible inclusion of some personal element:

1. Empowerment: an acknowledgement of expertise already possessed
2. Providing structured time for the trainee
3. Respect for the trainee as a fellow professional, from whom you expect professional standards
4. An awareness of their needs
5. To be accessible and available to the trainee as a counsellor as well as a mentor and assessor.

Indeed their view is that mentoring itself implies involvement with the learning progress of the student, whilst previous supervisory models in teacher training are seen as a lesser activity – merely 'keeping an eye' on the student.

Shaw[29] states clearly the case for inclusion of counselling skills in mentoring. In addition to the mentor's ability to use their own sound theoretical knowledge to help the mentee put knowledge into action, she sees a crucial aim of mentoring as one which moves the student into taking 'self responsibility' for their professional development. The foundation for this is the mentor's ability to enable the student to reflect on their practice, and engage in self-appraisal strategies. The approach has three parts:

1. Identifying and clarifying problem situations and unused opportunities
2. Goal setting – developing a more desirable scenario
3. Action – moving towards the preferred scenario.

Consideration of the potential conflicts inherent in the role of mentor, e.g. being a supportive friend and also an assessor, possible personality clashes between the mentor and student, and wider organizational issues which could hinder the learning process leads her to develop a model based on Egan's[30] ingredients of a skilled helper. Seen as essential are skills in communication, both verbal and non-verbal, in listening empathetically, confronting difficulties and employing negotiating skills to resolve them, and providing positive and negative feedback.

Education does not shy away from the word supervision, seeing it as a positive activity, not as overseeing or inspecting, but supporting and facilitating someone to become more effective. Supervisory skills are listed as:

Creating the appropriate climate, with trust and good communication
Reflecting on practice and performance review
Identifying learning needs, giving constructive feedback, and encouraging self evaluation
Supporting an enhanced understanding of the other's situation and their position in it
Setting goals and monitoring development.

Education also stresses the ongoing, continuing nature of mentoring, beyond that of inducting new teachers into the profession, and described by Kelly, Beck and Thomas[31] as a means of staff development. They see it as an effective means by which newly appointed head teachers, and lecturers in higher education, can gain an understanding of the structure and systems of their new organization, and also the underlying values existing within it, thus becoming more quickly and effectively established in their leadership role. This ongoing mentoring has the additional advantage of building a supportive structure throughout the organization; in addition, when mentors are assigned throughout the hierarchy, more individuals have the experience of both giving and receiving mentoring. The experience of these authors suggests that individuals are more likely to set themselves targets and change their behaviour as a result of feedback from a peer than from a line manager.

When mentoring is part of an organization's staff development programme, it provides staff with opportunities for:

Feedback on performance
Greater effectiveness in the workplace
Observing others as role models in work related activities
Personal support

and ensuring self review and appraisal in a professionally rigorous and challenging climate.

This finding is already embodied in the peer review structure of general practice, and introduces a theme concluded in the final chapter, that of the relationship between mentoring in general practice and the methods employed for the re-certification of practitioners. However, here, as in general practice, the authors do not address the more negative aspects of peer review, the risks of collusion, and those protection rackets which preserve the status quo.

Taylor[32] offered a small but important contribution to the concept of mentoring as a means of staff development. She perceived mentoring as an activity which would keep excellent practitioners in the classroom, providing sufficient stimulus and additional challenge to their own professional development to prevent their drift into managerial positions. This reinforces other views of mentors using their role to become themselves more reflective about their own practice, as well as keeping them abreast of new thinking and developments in practice. This concept of shared learning, in which the mentors themselves make professional gains through taking on the role, emerges sharply in Chapter 4.

Mentoring in education appears to confirm the themes identified in nursing – namely the integration of theory to practice, and support for taking on a new role. In addition, the pastoral aspect of mentoring finds a stronger voice, and a further component emerges – one which sees mentoring as a means of ensuring the professional development of all practitioners, mentors as well as mentees. These four components are taken forward and compared with accounts of mentoring in business organizations.

Part 4: Mentoring in business cultures

We look firstly at American business organizations, where the concept of mentoring seems never to have recovered from the impact of an article in the *Harvard Business Review*[33] entitled 'Everyone who makes it has a mentor'. This statement came in an interview with the chairman of a large company who disclosed that his rise to fame and fortune was in great part due to the patronage of an influential mentor early in his career, whose belief in 'giving young people their head' provided opportunities for developing responsibility and leadership.

This introduces an infinitely less altruistic theme, where mentoring is used as a promotional activity, the mentor acting as sponsor to ensure the career progression and success of an individual. A mentor appears as an influential person, someone who will argue the mentee's case with senior management for example. Rawlins and Rawlins[34] make some bold statements when advocating mentoring and 'networking' for professions, again based on a definition of mentoring to advance careers:

'mentors, teach, advise, open doors for, promote, cut red tape for [the protégé] . . . show the politics and subtleties of the job . . . thus helping them [protégés] to succeed'

and go on to state that:

'most important, mentors have skills, knowledge and power that protégés lack and need'
(p. 116).

Networking is placed within this context as a means of promoting helpful contacts for information, resources and career advancement, although we are exhorted to bear in mind that the strength of networking lies in mutual support rather than 'payback'.

Inasmuch as mentoring could be seen as an essential ingredient in a successful career, achieving this through the personal power and influence of the mentor rests uneasily with the notion of a shared learning process which fosters professional development. To restore the balance, a psycho-social component of mentoring, which relies heavily on theoretical constructs of adult growth and personality development, is central to much significant American writing on mentorship. This rests on concepts of developmental psychology, concepts which had a profound influence on Levinson *et al.*[35] referred to earlier in this chapter, who, in their study on the influence of mentors in the developing lives of 40 very different men, concluded that mentors were an integral part of the healthy development of a mature personality. Conversely, Fury[36] used Levinson's psycho-social definition of a mentor as a wise, influential parent, and interviewed 100 men and women in middle management positions on their experience of such a mentor. Only one person reported having had one.

Examples of mentors at work in British business suggest that the power of the mentor to progress your career is less blatant, although advice on a future career path appears as a core aim. In the six examples described in a recent Incomes Data Service report,[37] a 'culturization' of the mentee into the company appeared consistently as a core aim, together with personal and career development, and networking opportunities. Whilst all six companies described schemes which focused on the young entrant, Price Waterhouse gave an interesting and relevant account of the need, in a market which reduces opportunities for new entrants to become partners of the firm, to encourage senior members to take on different, wider roles in the company, not necessarily promotion. This was an additional stated aim of their mentoring scheme. Whilst mentors offered the individual objective advice, increasing their confidence and building skills for present and future roles, the following company benefits also came out of the individual mentoring relationship:

- Helps succession planning
- Raises motivation
- Can aid employee retention
- Is a cost effective method of staff development.

It was interesting to read these, for, quite unknowingly, the original funding proposal submitted for the mentor scheme described here had been placed before the health authority in 1994, and had set very similar objectives, whilst stressing the importance of an available mentor for established, mature practitioners.

Whilst the power based interpretation of business mentoring leaves it outside mentoring models in the professions of nursing and teaching, business has addressed the application of mentoring to the role of women in business.

Women, sex and mentors

The literature points to two major problems in the formation of mentoring relationships for women: the lack of women in high managerial positions to act as mentors to younger women, and the potential sexual problems in male mentor/female protégée relationships.

Sheehy[38] asserted that almost without exception the women who gained recognition in their careers were at some point nurtured by a mentor, whilst Kanter[39] found that women who failed to progress did so because they were without mentors to provide sponsorship. Hennig and Jardim[40] concluded from their study of 25 top women executives that women wanting to succeed must look for someone in a more senior position to advise and support their advancement, although other studies counter this, concluding that for women, the presence of a mentor in one's career was not a critical variable to succeed.

Do women do better with women mentors? The influence of initial role models for career women is discussed by some authors, who consider the likelihood of career-orientated mothers providing a role model for their daughters which then enables them to progress more easily in their own career.[41,42] This theme is relevantly described in the reporting of a mentoring in the council offices of the London Borough of Brent.[43] The mentor scheme was devised to address the under-representation of women in their higher management grades and, to rectify this, mentoring was explicitly targeted at female junior and middle managers. The scheme defined a mentor as being a transitional figure, someone who would help you move forward and upward on the career ladder, but their mentor team had to include men because of insufficient women in managerial positions available to take on the role. Mentees working with a woman mentor found them particularly helpful in formulating survival strategies, while those working with a male mentor felt this added a different, unquantifiable dimension to the process, but not a negative one. In reporting this study, the final evaluation showed that gender was of far less importance than the individual attributes of the mentor, a finding replicated in our own study.

Women, then, need mentors who can provide good role models as much as anything else, but the scarcity of women in appropriate positions to do this is a factor that works against women acting as mentors to other women. This would avoid the sexual aspect that would appear from the literature as being an almost inevitable outcome of male/female pairings. Philips-Jones[44] found that the number of cross-sex dyads in mentoring relationships which developed romantic or sexual overtones exceeded her expectations, and Sheehy[45] warns:

'when a man becomes interested in guiding and advising younger women there is usually an erotic interest that goes along with it' (p.189).

Although other authors support the view of romantic liaisons arising from male/female mentor partnerships, there is little said of the potentially romantic outcomes when the woman is older than her male mentor. Levinson[46] describes mentoring which sets out to gain sexual favours as 'flawed mentoring', although it is not clear whether the mentor pair them-selves see this additional component as a flaw, or whether Levinson has assumed it to be so.

Apart from aspects of age and sex, there does appear to be a lack of female mentors. In general practice, there are more male mentors than women – in our own mentoring team of 20, there are only three women. In business organizations, three factors emerge which are seen to explain the lack of female mentors:

1. Little recognition of women's skill and achievement in their orga-nizations – women have to be more than better than men to be acknowledged.
2. The Queen Bee syndrome – successful younger women are threats to older established women who will therefore do nothing to support them.
3. Too few women in senior positions to take on female protégées.

Whilst there are some obvious departures from the mentor models described in nursing and education, there is some overlap. The business literature does support the view that mentoring is an activity defined pri-marily by the context in which it takes place, and in British business there is some indication that mentoring can be used flexibly to reflect economic change, and meet the changing needs of the workforce. Business mentor-ing is similarly interested in career advancement, but it appears as an entity in itself. Personal growth, if it occurs, is not a stated aim, but a side product.

Patronage is readily acknowledged as a means of gaining power. This is not to imply that other organizations stand apart from such sordid enter-prise; indeed general practice maintains in large measure a system of net-working and patronage, but it is not seen in conjunction with a mentor's role.

So, one variant in the weighting appears. In developing a holistic mentor model for general practice, a mentor was envisaged as someone who, through offering a consistent, supportive relationship, *empowers* the mentee to take charge of their own life. In some business organizations, it is the *mentor's power* that advances the mentee to a higher position in their career – a 'fast-tracking' device. It is not clear whether the mentee then embarks on the transitional journey enabling him or her to achieve the maturity to execute the task.

From the business arena come some interesting data on the needs of women, and gender issues in the mentoring relationship. As there is grow-ing interest in hospital medicine in mentoring networks which advance women's careers, particularly in consultant-level appointments, this is discussed further in Chapter 8.

Certainly the sexual implications of cross-sex mentoring can be located in the anecdotal experience of male GP trainers working with younger female trainees. It is an aspect well documented in the therapeutic profes-sions, where the therapeutic relationship raises awareness of inappropriate sexual counter-transference. In the final part of the review, the therapeutic disciplines are explored – not for examples of sexuality in the helping relationship, but instead to compare the model of professional supervision in the helping professions with that of the mentor.

Part 5: Supervision in the helping professions

Definitions of supervision

The dictionary definitions support the common view of supervision as an activity which oversees the actions of another, and whilst there is a reassuring element of directing and guiding, equally an autocratic aspect is implied.

These images were confirmed in the pilot questionnaire which formed part of the first phase of this research into the development of mentoring, when 40 doctors were asked for immediate responses to what the word 'mentoring' meant to them, and what the word 'supervision' conjured up. Supervision was seen as being directive, at times welcome, but on the whole negative, with supervisors being viewed as authoritarian in their role.

As someone who had begun their professional life in psychology, and trained as a psychotherapist, supervision had quite a different meaning. It was a positive intervention closely resembling the concept of supervision in higher education described earlier in this chapter. Yet in reviewing the literature of the helping professions, there was a startling absence of explanations about the nature of that difference. This in itself was interesting, for it implies that authors (themselves practitioners) take for granted that the reader knows it to be a positive and necessary part of professional practice, and so focus primarily on exploring the complexities of the process.

Nevertheless, definitions of supervision are given, and appear somewhat more assured than those ascribed to mentoring. For example Hess[47] provides a confident and concise definition:

'a quintessential, interpersonal interaction with the general goal that one person, the supervisor, meets with another – the supervisee – in an effort to make the latter more effective in helping people'

and Loganbill *et al.*[48] similarly define it as:

'an intensive, interpersonally focused, one to one relationship in which one person is designated to facilitate the development of therapeutic competence in the other person.'

These are both American definitions. In Britain, the 1950s saw the development of teaching and learning in social work practice, and in one of the first British books on student supervision Young[49] bases the supervisory task on a hierarchical relationship of the supervisor as teacher and the student as learner. This appears as the pattern of the time, and echoes current theory-to-practice mentoring models in nursing.

But Gardiner[50] is critical of what later developed, which he succinctly describes as 'concept leakage'. As it developed, the supervision process used the same concepts underlying traditional one-to-one casework (therapeutic) practice, mixing these with a didactic model of teaching. This meant that, in addition to the *educative* component, there was an overt assumption that the *emotional* growth of the student was part and parcel of supervision, so that the psycho-analytic model of the analyst/analysand, or patient/therapist relationship was 'leaked' into the supervisory relationship.

Here, it seems, began the continuing confusion between supervising the professional task of a worker, and giving them (at times without their explicit consent) 'personal therapy'. This aspect has many supporters in general practice, similarly concerned about concept leakage, and fearful that mentoring might become (or already is) personal therapy. When verbalized, this concern seems to suffer from confusion and ambivalence in equal measure. It is much harder for doctors to clearly define and distinguish therapy from counselling, and other forms of helping intervention, as very few of them have been formally trained in either. At the same time, doctors encounter an element of 'counselling' within the consultation, so that they feel confident and familiar with using these skills, perceiving themselves, often accurately, as an occasional counsellors to their patients. Yet these same skills, applied differently, to peers not patients, strike dread in their hearts. Then it seems that basic counselling is metamorphosed into therapy, and must be avoided. So is the shying away from entering the personal, inner world of another person (not a patient) explained by a flawed assumption as to what personal therapy is, or leaking concepts?

Gardiner[51] is particularly helpful here, being critical of a style of supervision in which the supervisee's learning and development is seen as synonymous with emotional growth. The problems he or she encounters in the learning are pathologized, and little account is taken of the difference in learning styles and preferences of the person being supervised, and little attention paid to the educative element of the relationship. Instead, the supervisee is treated as a passive client, with the supervisor focusing on feelings, rather than integrating sufficiently the adult learning processes which encourage the supervisee to be active in their supervision, and thereby the professional development.

This criticism clearly encapsulates the need for boundaries in the mentor's role, discussed in the following chapter, and referred to by other authors writing from within the helping professions. Atherton[52] is also clear that therapy and counselling have no place in supervision:

'I am not really interested in the feelings or problems of the staff member himself – except in so far as he needs to be able to contain them and resolve them in such a way as to free him to work effectively' [with clients] (p.127).

However, this does not imply that the supervisor is simply a teacher. Truax and Karkhuff[53] state that the supervisor needs to possess the classic three-fold qualities of the counsellor and to be able to adopt them as principles in supervision – the qualities of empathy, warmth and genuineness. Kurpius[54] also includes 'personal and emotional development' (p. 65) as one of the supervisor's functions, and states that supervisors need to provide for supervisees the same conditions for therapeutic change they offer their clients, so that their supervisees can become more open and less defensive. To provide this supportive yet challenging component, consistently quoted as a crucial element in both mentoring and supervision, it would seem that both mentors and supervisors would do well to possess and use skills traditionally associated with counselling.

How do supervisors achieve this, whilst at the same time avoiding the unhelpful aspect of 'concept leakage' referred to earlier, where the supervisee is steered towards the passive role of client, rather than active learner? Obviously, clear boundaries have to be constantly observed between the different aspects of the supervisory task. One way of keeping boundaries is through the use of contracts, which make clear the purpose and content of supervision:

'An explicit contract is a statement by both supervisor and staff member about the objectives and topics of their particular supervision sessions, and what each will do in order to meet these objectives'[55] (p. 35).

Contracts, it seems, not only delineate boundaries, but are useful in demonstrating that the supervisee has equal responsibility in contributing to the effectiveness of the supervisory relationship. It makes clear both what is on offer from the supervisor, and what is requested from the supervisee. It ensures that both people are talking about the same thing, and can incorporate practical aspects such as protected time, venue for meetings, the priorities for discussion, and reporting back.

Unlike the mentoring literature, which made little explicit reference to the chronological and professional age of the mentee, there is a suggestion here that the contract needs to reflect the 'age and stage' of the supervisee. In the initial phase of their practice, the supervisee may be closer to the student role and require the focus of supervision to be geared towards training and teaching, whilst experienced practitioners will consult with their supervisor, who is neither a trainer nor a manager, on the issues they themselves have identified for exploration.

A more familiar word – consultation – is offered by Brown[56] and Kadushin.[57] They share a similar definition of consultation as being an interactional helping process, a series of sequential steps taken to achieve an objective via an interpersonal relationship. One participant – the consultant – has greater knowledge, skill and expertise in a particular function. The consultee has encountered a problem or situation in his/her job which requires the extra knowledge and skill of the consultant and its amelioration. Kadushin distinguishes consultation from other helping, interpersonally based activities such as therapy by virtue of its problem-solving focus – it is clearly job related. Consultation, then, seems not to concern itself with emotional growth, but with problem solving. Consultation used in this context then would appear to have a relationship with mentoring, but does supervision offer a closer model?

Hawkins and Shohet,[58] in providing an extensive overview of the purpose and activity of supervision, set out the belief on which supervision in the helping professions is predicated – namely that professional helpers are involved at the coal face of working with people who are distressed, ill, or in some way emotionally dishevelled, and are therefore exposed to negative attacks from their patients or clients. These powerful experiences are potentially disabling and damaging to the worker, and can best be survived through the strength of a supervisory relationship. The role of a supervisor is not to reassure, but to allow the emotional disturbance encountered in the work to be re-experienced within a safe setting – so that supervision acts as a container. By reflecting on such encounters, the projective mechanism of blaming others for one's failures and setbacks is avoided, enabling the worker to learn from negative experiences.

The authors set out three components which they see as being incorporated in the role of the supervisor: an educational component, a supportive component, and a managerial component.

As an educator, the supervisor offers the opportunity for reflection and exploration of work, in order to understand their client better, and become more aware of their own responses and reactions to the dynamics of their helping relationship. The consequences of their intervention are compared and contrasted with other ways in which the work could have been approached, thereby offering learning from the work base.

As a supporter, the supervisor increases the supervisee's awareness of how their work with clients affects them personally, and helps them to deal with their reactions. This is seen as essential if the worker is not to become over-identified with their clients, and be drained by the emotional demands made upon them, and equally to avoid the unhelpful strategy of defending against being affected by them.

The authors use an interesting analogy here of the British miners, who in 1920 fought for the right to wash off the day's filth and grime from their colliery work in their bosses' time, rather than taking it home with them, and state that the supportive element of supervision is equivalent of 'pit-head' time.

The managerial component is the quality control function held by the supervisor, which ensures that the standards of the agency are upheld, and that the work of the supervisee falls within defined ethical standards.

In the therapeutic disciplines, supervision is 'built in', part of the stated requirement of the task – unlike mentoring, which for many organizations is still an 'optional extra'. Furthermore, in psychotherapy and counselling, the therapist is not allowed to practise without evidence of being supervised. This implies that supervision is fundamental to good practice, and some authors address the harm arising to both the professional practitioner, and their client, when supervision is absent. Kurpius[59] states that a lack of supervision leads to staleness, rigidity and defensiveness in the worker, and its continuing absence is a contributory factor to job stress and burnout. Supervision is seen as a necessary activity for all workers, throughout the organization.

This integrative approach avoids the belief that helpers are problem free and only patients or clients are needy. This introduces a very relevant concept for general practice, that of the wounded healer. What is it that motivates individuals to become helpers, of healers to heal? Is it in part their need to work out their own unresolved difficulties about caring and being cared for, and/or a need for power over others, in the disguise of the helper? If the dimension of power is to be used constructively, it needs to be openly acknowledged. Similarly, when wounded healers share their experience of wounding, they find it enhances their ability to care, and provides valuable learning for colleague-healers. But, as we have stated, medicine shies away from such openness, fearing loss of status. Dass and Gorman[60] state the infallible doctor's dilemma very precisely:

'Many helpers, when they themselves are suffering are incapable of accepting support, or at least receiving it easily. Yet they may be impatient with those they're working with for

not accepting aid or counsel readily enough. Chances are – if you can't accept help you can't really give it' (p. 129).

The implication is that by receiving consistent supervision the worker is enabled to go about their work unencumbered by the residue of negative emotional transactions, whilst learning how to receive, use and value the support of others. A further spin-off is that they themselves more readily offer support to others.

But is it always so splendid? Apparently not, and Shohet and Hawkins[61] tell us four reasons why supervision might not be so effective:

1. Previous experience of supervision: if it has been bad the supervisee is made wary; if good, then the supervisee might feel that no other supervisor lives up to their previous one
2. Personal inhibition: the threat of a searching one-to-one relationship, of being put 'on the spot', having to account for one's behaviour
3. Transference in the supervisory relationship: projecting on to the supervisor critical, negative images, commonly those of a critical parent
4. Organizational blocks: the fear that a lack of confidentiality might block career progression, or affect one's standing in the professional community.

Whilst supervision, like mentoring, has a preference for one-to-one individual supervision models, it has two additional models: group supervision and peer supervision.

In group supervision, the supervisor leads a group whose members have the same work experience, share similar conceptual frameworks, but otherwise have different ranges of skill, experience and age. Their shared experience of the task is used as the learning base, with members taking it in turns to quite formally and carefully present a case study. Advantages to this method are seen in the ways in which the members themselves contribute to the supervisory process, and widen dimensions of insight and available expertise, with economies of scale.

The disadvantages of group supervision are eloquently and humorously described by Houston[62] who writes of the competitive games and traps set by group members for each other. 'Measuring cocks', based on 'my work's better than yours', and 'look how good I am' is one of them. 'Ain't it awful' games are played to reassure members that their task is impossible, which serves to reinforce their sense of powerlessness at work and the uselessness of attempting anything. A skilled supervisor to act as leader is essential to group supervision, which does not entirely replace individual supervision sessions, but is provided in addition.

Whilst group supervision seems to offer a relevant framework for supervising the work of a team of mentors, and would have the advantage of economy of scale, particularly in general practice where budgets are tightly constrained, it loses the central one-to-one relationship of a mentor working individually with a mentee. Did the second model – peer supervision – move any closer to mentoring?

Peer supervision originated in humanistic psychotherapy, where practitioners are dedicated to the concept of continuous supervision throughout professional life, incorporating the use of peers for reflection and analysis of work. Hawkins and Shoet[63] give an account of a peer triad, a psychiatrist, psychotherapist, and clinical psychologist. One person will take turns at providing 40 minutes of supervision for each of the other two, with time for feedback at the end of the session. Although economy of time and resources are again an obvious advantage, in the helping professions peer supervision is used mainly as a model for learning how to supervise, and in practice suffers from the difficulty of getting three people together in one place, at one time, on a consistent basis. Without an identified leader who sits outside the discussion and monitors the structure, it is easier for all three parties to overrun their allotted time, as everyone is in the same position of wanting time and attention for their agenda. But the greatest risk is of collusion, where colleagues avoid 'rocking the boat' and usefully challenging each other, choosing to maintain a comfortable, easy atmosphere, offering only reassurance of the rightness of their ways.

Summary

Overall, the unifying theme of mentoring lies in its context, not its definition. Mentoring models in the different professions are shaped, it seems, by the context of the work setting. The objectives of the mentoring intervention are linked to perceived organizational needs, and to the task in which the organization is engaged.

Four common objectives of mentoring are drawn from the literature:

1. Mentoring assists in the application and integration of 'institutionally based' learning to the reality of professional practice
2. Mentoring supports and assists the transitional process of taking up a new role in the workplace, of becoming a fully-fledged professional
3. Mentoring can bring benefits to an organization by promoting a supportive structure for staff development
4. Mentoring supports continuing personal and professional growth.

To what extent were these objectives currently located in the field of general practice mentoring? Certainly some similarities between mentor roles in other professions and existing roles in general practice became more sharply defined. It appeared that the first two objectives were already met in general practice, and very successfully. The GP trainer is placed in a classic mentor role, being a senior practitioner assisting a young practitioner in their transitional journey towards full professional adulthood. Trainers help their registrars to put theory into the reality of practice, integrate new learning, and assist the process of what the American literature refers to as 'acculturation' – being inducted into, and becoming part of, the culture of general practice.

The legacy of the medical apprenticeship model does, it seems, leave medical practitioners with an innate recognition that their transitional journey from student to master will be littered with trials of inner strength, and other obstacles. Perhaps for this reason, Young Practitioner groups thrive in general practice, offering a further potential source of mentoring. The support of one's peers could be extremely useful in the transitional process of moving from apprentice (trainee) to journeyman (young practitioner) and finally to master (principal). However, informal evidence suggests that the usefulness of these groups varies. Whilst some do offer potential mentor-type support, others are purely social, making the provision of such support a hit-and-miss affair.

Comparing similarities in mentoring between general practice and other professions enabled differences to become more clearly etched. Women trying to make it to the top in medicine frequently face the same isolation and repression experienced by their counterparts in the business world, and likewise lack suitable mentors. However, unlike the world of business, there is little hierarchical career progression in general practice; where it exists, it is self-directed. If GP mentors were to promote the career progression of their mentees, it would be indirectly, through enabling them to make decisions which widened rather than heightened his or her career, rather than being in a position to directly promote their mentee's interests. And, given the relationship between the (then) demoralized climate of general practice and the rise of interest in mentorship, it seemed preferable, and sensible, to leave aside the formal appraisal, or assessing element linked to mentoring in higher education, so that mentors were not viewed as formal evaluators of competence to practice.

Another difference was related to professional age. The target of mentoring in other professions is the young practitioner. Those entering a new profession are, of course, likely to use their mentors well, initially to their individual advantage, but eventually to benefit their organization. As we have seen, the nursing profession used mentors to improve the retention rate of expensively trained practitioners, and retention and recruitment is today a strong argument for the development of general practice mentoring. Yet transitional stages occur throughout life and, given the context of this study, it was important to make mentors available to all doctors, at whatever age and stage of their professional life.

Finally, the comparison revealed a critical conceptual difference. In none of the professions explored was the mentor seen as a crisis counsellor, someone who appeared in times of trouble and then departed. Mentors were part of the ongoing life of the organization, a steady and continuing thread in the fabric of professional induction and development. Transition is not to be confused with crisis, for although the process of moving from one state of being to another can be accompanied by a sense of destabilization and confusion, there is not the same degree of overwhelming chaos which renders coping strategies redundant. Inevitably, and rightly, there are times when people in organizations turn to their mentor when in crisis and, usually, if their crisis develops, are referred to more appropriate sources of help, for instance marital therapy. The far more common picture is of mentoring as an ongoing developmental activity. It appears as a place to go and formulate strategies for overcoming obstacles which lie on the path of progression, and to share the triumphs of overcoming them, or simply to make realistic plans for one's professional future life. The following chapter will tell of the importance of distinguishing between working within an organizational climate of crisis and working with an individual in crisis.

These differences served to focus the formulation of a mentor model for general practice on outcomes which matched the last two objectives emerging from the literature review. Firstly, drawn from higher education and British business was a macro-view of mentoring as an 'in-house' support structure for staff development, with the potential benefit to the medical profession as a whole. Secondly, from the supervision model of the helping professions came a convergence of their professional beliefs and practice which gave prominence to individual support to practitioners to encourage their continuing personal and professional growth.

Ignorance, as all educated people know, is bliss. What you don't know, you don't have to think about, let alone act upon. When learning from the literature on mentoring was applied to the context of general practice, it indicated on the one hand, that the window of opportunity was wide open. A broader understanding of how mentors functioned elsewhere was invaluable in defining what general practice mentors might do. The research proposal, which asked for sufficient funding to implement the mentoring concept, to review its progress, and evaluate its outcome, was successful – Allah, it seemed, in this respect being one and the same as the Accursed One, and unable to return to the task which the Devil had spoiled, was prepared at least to fund a product designed to help men (and women) and make things easier for them.

But the ravines still existed. From where would come the sales force? In a profession known to be demoralized, stressed, and overworked, how was such a role as this to be effectively 'sold' to practitioners? Who would voluntarily risk yet more contamination from the distress of others, particularly as these 'others' are peers, people just like us, lacking the benefit of being classed as a 'patient' and therefore more easily placed at a safe distance from the self?

Furthermore, the review of mentoring in other professions did not set out specifically to identify common attributes of mentors which would enable the objective of the relationship to be achieved, although they are referred to frequently in later chapters. Nevertheless, it was difficult to escape the conclusion that mentors are exemplars of professional practice, persons of obvious, outstanding integrity, possessing almost magical skills in communication and problem solving. The objectives of modern mentoring have strayed somewhat from those on offer in ancient Greece. Still, it seems aspiring mentors take history and myth seriously, looking back at Mentor as an inspiring role model, and continually seeking to emulate his goddess-given qualities. Who amongst the professional community would identify these aspects in themselves? Equally concerning was the nagging doubt that those who might so confidently declare themselves, and come forward, are likely to be the least appropriate personalities to undertake the role.

These considerations emphasized the critical overlap between the formulation and implementation stages of planned development. The role of a general practice mentor had to be formulated in such a way that made it desirable, and obviously manageable to potential mentors – both in its description and, later, in practice. Unless the concept was introduced in a way which meant that potential mentors could quickly identify with the proposed new role, and imagine themselves working with it in the field, we would not recruit anyone willing to test the idea, and the window of opportunity would be slammed shut.

Like crows gathering over the stubble fields of autumn, those cynical of the proposed mentoring scheme watched and waited, anticipating the downfall of another good idea, while those intent upon its implementation gathered strength for its introduction.

The Hippocratic Oath

I swear by Apollo the leader, by Aesculapius, by Health and all the powers of healing, and call to witness all the gods and goddesses that I may keep this Oath and Promise to the best of my ability and judgement.

I will pay the same respect to my master in the Science as to my parents and share my life with him and pay all my debts to him. I will regard his sons as my brothers and teach them the Science, if they desire to learn it, without fee or contract. I will hand on my precepts lectures and all other learning to my sons, to those of my master, and to those pupils duly apprenticed and sworn, and to none other.

I will use my power to help the sick to the best of my ability and judgement; I will abstain from harming or wronging any man by it.

I will not give a fatal draught to anyone if I am asked, nor will I suggest any such thing. Neither will I give a woman means to procure an abortion.

I will be chaste and religious in my life and my practice.

I will not cut, even for the stone, but I will leave such procedures to the practitioners of that craft.

Whenever I go into a house, I will go to help the sick and never with the intention of doing harm or injury. I will not abuse my position to indulge in sexual contracts with the bodies of women or of men, whether they be freemen or slaves.

Whatever I see or hear, professionally or privately, which ought not to be divulged, I will keep secret and tell no one.

If therefore I observe this Oath and do not violate it, may I prosper both in my life and in my profession, earning good repute among all men for all time. If I transgress and forswear this Oath, may my lot be otherwise.

Cited in the *Cambridge Illustrated History: Medicine*, edited Roy Porter, p. 59

References

1 Homer 1969 *The Odyssey*. Simon and Shuster, New York
2 Sutton V. 1995 Medicine in the Greek world – 800–50BC. In *The Western Medical Tradition – 800BC to AD1800* (eds Conrad I.L., Neve M., Sutton V., Porter R. and Wear A.) Cambridge University Press, Cambridge
3 Sivin, N. 1995 Text and experience in classical Chinese medicine. In *Knowledge and the Scholarly Medical Traditions* (ed. Bates D.) Cambridge University Press, Cambridge
4 Lipsey R. 1988 *An Art of our Own: The Spiritual in 20th Century Art*. Shambhala Publications, Boston, Massachusetts

5 Lawrence S.C. 1985 Desirous of improvements in medicine: pupils and practitioners in the Medical Societies at Guy's and St. Bartholomew's Hospitals, 1795–1815. *Bulletin of the History of Medicine*, **59**(1), 89–104

6 Silvermann M.E. 1993 James Bovell: a remarkable 19th century physician and the forgotten mentor of William Osler. *Canadian Medical Association Journal*, **148**(6), 953–7

7 Barondess J.A. 1997 On mentoring. *Journal of the Royal Society of Medicine*, **90**, June, 347–9

8 Op. cit

9 Merriam S. 1983 Mentors and proteges: a critical review of the literature. *Adult Education Quarterly*, **33**, 161–73

10 Carruthers J. 1993 In *Return of the Mentor – Strategies for Workplace Learning* (eds Caldwell B. and Carter E.A.) Falmer Press, London

11 Carmin C.N. 1988 Issues on research in mentoring: definitional and methodological. *International Journal of Mentoring*, **2-2**, 9–13

12 Ibid

13 Philips-Jones L. 1982 *Mentors and Proteges*. Arbour House, New York

14 Levinson K, Darrow C., Klein E., Levinson M and McKee B. 1978 *Seasons of a Man's Life*. Alfred A. Knopf, New York

15 Winnicott, D. 1978 *Playing and Reality*. Pelican, London

16 Darling, L.A. 1984 What do nurses want in a mentor? *Journal of Nursing Administration*, **14**(10), 42–4

17 Jacobi M. 1991 Mentoring and undergraduate academic success: a literature review. *Review of Educational Research*, **61**(4), 505–32

18 Kramer M. 1974 *Reality Shock*. Mosby, St. Louis

19 Ibid

20 Morle K.M.F. 1990 Mentorship – is it a case of the Emperor's New Clothes or a rose by any other name? *Nurse Education Today*, **10**, 66–9

21 Chickerella B.G. and Lutz W.J. 1981 Professional nurturance preceptorships for undergraduate nursing. *American Journal of Nursing*, **81**(1), 17–119

22 Armitage P. and Burnard P. 1991 Mentors or preceptors? Narrowing the theory practice gap. *Nurse Education Today*, **11**, 225–9

23 Gerrish C. Fumbling along. *Nursing Times*, **86**(30)

24 Morton-Cooper A. and Palmer A. 1993 *Mentoring and Preceptorship – A Guide to Support Roles in Clinical Practice*. Blackwell Science, UK

25 Ibid

26 Wilkin M. 1992 *Mentoring in Schools*. Kogan Page, London

27 Black D. and Booth M. 1992 Structured mentoring. In *Mentoring in Schools*, ibid

28 Hurst B, and Wilkin M. 1992 Guidelines for mentors. In *Mentoring in Schools*, ibid

29 Shaw R. 1992 Can mentoring raise achievement in schools? In *Mentoring in Schools*, ibid

30 Egan G. 1990 *The Skilled Helper – A Systematic Approach to Effective Helping*. Brooks Cole Company, Pacific Grove CA

31 Kelly M., Beck T. and apThomas J. 1992 Mentoring as staff development. In *Mentoring in Schools*, ibid

32 Taylor, S. 1986 Mentors: who are they and what are they doing? *Thrust for Education Leadership*, **15**(7), 247–51

33 Lundin F., Clements G. and Perkins D. 1978 Mentoring relationships: everyone who makes it has a mentor. *Harvard Business Review*, **7.8**, July, 89–101

34 Rawlins M. and Rawlins L. 1983 Mentoring and networking for helping professionals. *Personnel and Guidance Journal*, **62**(2), October, 116–19

35 Ibid

36 Fury K. 1979 Mentor mania. *Savvy*, December, **427**, 119–21

37 IDS Study 613 *Mentoring Schemes*. November 1996. Incomes Data Services Ltd, 193 St. John's Street, London EC1V 4LS

38 Sheehy G. 1976 The mentor connection: the secret link in the successful woman's life. *New York Magazine*, 33–9

39 Kanter R.M. 1977 *Men and Women of the Corporation*. Basic Books, New York

40 Henning M. and Jardim A. 1977 *The Managerial Woman.* Doubleday, New York
41 Almquist E. and Angrist S. 1971 *Role Model Influences on College Women's Career Aspirations: The Professional Woman.* Shenkman, Boston MA
42 Rapaport R. and Rapaport R. 1971 Early and later experiences as determinants of adult behaviour: married women's family and career patterns. *British Journal of Sociology,* **22**, 16–30
43 IDS Study, ibid.
44 Philips-Jones L. 1982 ibid
45 Ibid
46 Ibid
47 Hess A.K. 1980 *Psychotherapy Supervision: Theory Research and Practice.* Wiley, New York
48 Loganbill C., Hardy E. and Delworth O. 1982 Supervision: a conceptual model. *The Counselling Psychologist USA,* **10**(1), 3–42
49 Young P. 1967 *The Student and Supervision in Social Work Education.* Routledge and Kegan Paul, London
50 Gardiner J. 1989 *The Anatomy of Supervision: Developing Learning and Professional Competence for Social Work Students.* Society for Research into Higher Education. Open University Press, Milton Keynes
51 Ibid
52 Atherton J. 1986 *Professional Supervision in Group Care.* Tavistock Publications, London
53 Truax C. and Karkhuff R. 1967 *Towards Effective Counselling and Psychotherapy.* Aldine, Chicago IL
54 Ibid
55 Ibid
56 Brown, S. 1967 Pragmatic notes on community consultation with agencies. *Community Health Journal,* **3**, 399–405
57 Kadushin A. 1977 *Consultation in Social Work.* Columbia University Press, New York
58 Hawkins P. and Shoet R. 1989 *Supervision in the Helping Professions.* Open University Press, Milton Keynes
59 Ibid
60 Dass, R. and ad Gorman P. 1985 *How Can I Help?* Rider, London
61 Ibid
62 Houseton G. 1985 Games people play in supervision. *Social Work Today,* **33**(11), 13–21
63 Op cit
64 Heron J. 1975 *Criteria for Evaluating Growth Movement.* University of Surrey, Guildford

3

Ideas into reality: From formulation to implementation

'theatetus' – mental midwifery – bringing into the light of day ideas which are latent in the mind

(Plato)

This chapter is in four parts. This first part describes the formulation of a holistic model of mentoring, and comments on professional conversations which influenced its design. The resulting structure and administrative framework for a mentor scheme is then outlined. Part 2 introduces a strategy, called the Reflective Cycle, designed to aid the establishment of mentor–mentee relationships, and seen as an important tool in the mentoring process. Part 3 provides a picture of these ideas being tested with intending mentors via a series of introductory workshops. It tells how the participants of the workshops, all intending mentors, responded to using the ideas, before a summary which reflects on relevant themes emerging from the workshop experience. In the fourth and final section of the chapter, a descriptive account of the early experience of the mentor team when putting the model to use, and how the model worked in practice, is given. Finally, the learning of the implementation phase is summarized to show its place in the emerging framework which established a structure for the ongoing South Thames Mentor Scheme.

Part 1: Formulating a mentor model

Personal influences

Reviewing the literature gave greater credence to my own developing concept of a model of mentoring for general practice which was 'holistic'.[1] Holistic implies an intervention that holds together the three classic components of mentoring that emerged from the review, and clearly distinguish mentoring from other forms of helping intervention:

Personal support
Continuing education
Professional development.

The mentor would afford equal weighting between these elements, helping their mentee to manage transitional states, acquire or integrate new learning, and maximize their potential to become fulfilled and effective practitioners. The model would have, as its first objective, encouraging and supporting personal and professional growth, through a continuing relationship. If this could be developed, it would offer the further benefit of changing the organizational climate of medicine, by providing a supportive structure for professional development.

From these, and other considerations belonging to the pre-pilot phase of study, the definition and task of potential mentors in the South Thames (West) scheme was drafted, and reads:

'A mentor is a senior practitioner, or a respected peer, who offers, through an ongoing professional relationship with his or her mentee, opportunities to develop, stimulate, and maintain their professional development by:

> *addressing current professional concerns*
> *identifying further learning needs*
> *providing space and time to reflect on, and evaluate the professional task*
> *identifying blocks or hindrances to the professional well-being of their mentee*
> *offering help with career appraisal and development'*[2]

More personal influences on the formulation of this model came from previous experience in the field, and formal and informal exchanges with practitioners and colleagues. These, like a good mentor, shaped the emerging concept and structure of holistic mentoring, albeit at times unknowingly.

My role as Educational Adviser in general practice, whilst something of a balancing act between academic professional education and pragmatic involvement, is not a confining one. Working alongside medical colleagues in primary and secondary care, both at home and abroad, on a variety of educational ventures, provides valuable opportunities to talk, reflect, and share experiences of working life. After 1995, and the implementation of the new contract, these informal, but professional conversations frequently turned to the state of general practice, vividly described by one colleague as

'a beleaguered profession mourning its lost self image'.[3]

These conversations were typified by an evident eagerness on the part of the practitioners to share with me their working experience, to seek some measure of support for difficult encounters and events, to search out suggestions for change, even at times to ask for advice, although I was outside the profession.

I began to see in these encounters a microcosm of the isolation and lack of support felt by many doctors within their professional community. Although most doctors were working within group practices, surrounded by their peers, they felt 'on the edges' – a description I personally identified with, working as I did on the margins of a profession, being neither insider nor total outsider.

These discussions were more personal echoes of the findings of numerous research studies reported in the professional literature which gave evidence of stress and demoralization in general practice and, putting the discussion experience and reading together, served to reinforce my perception of the need to design a mentor scheme in such a way as to both increase the wellbeing of individual doctors, and hold the capacity to become an 'in-house' supportive framework. But there was a problem.

I had been a mentor in a university setting and, before moving into education, a previous career in psychotherapy had made me familiar with a model of clinical supervision, both being supervised myself and working as a supervisor to others (a model closely akin to classic mentoring). Yet, talking with doctors revealed no resemblance between my own experience and understanding of mentor roles, and their own concept of mentoring. Those who did have some idea of what a mentor should do described an activity which, to my eyes and ears, was more closely related to limited educational supervision, whilst others had no idea, but sensed mentoring was 'a good thing'. I had a strong impression of a profession reaching towards something called mentoring, without quite knowing what it was.

This made me increasingly thoughtful about my own understanding of a mentor's role. Were these doctors simply misinformed or, as the literature suggested, were they in the process of finding a style of mentoring that would fit their particular need and context? Equally, did my previous knowledge and experience bias my interpretation of what constituted effective mentoring activity? After all, doctors fall into the trap of 'knowing best' (although at times they do) and prescribing for their patient not what the patient needs, but what the doctor thinks is good for them. How could I be reasonably sure that I was not about to do the same?

Professional influences

To further ensure that the holistic model was, as far as is possible, responsive to actual need, and would be positively received by general practitioners, it was necessary to do further work; so, to support the formal and informal evidence gathered thus far, two small, qualitative studies were undertaken. One study, which used an administered questionnaire to a convenience sample of 52 GPs, sought firstly for further information about the need (or otherwise) for professional support. This enquired about their current support systems, whom they turned to for support, whether they preferred to keep their own counsel when faced with troubling professional events, and whether they felt they gave out more support to others than they themselves received. The response to this latter question showed all respondents feeling that they gave out more support than they received, and indicated various ways in which they would welcome more support for themselves.

As there appeared to be lack of clarity about the different activities of mentoring and supervision, the second dimension of the questionnaire tried to shed light on this, by asking the respondent for a spontaneous reply to what the words 'mentor' and 'supervisor' conjured up. This showed that mentoring carried a more attractive image than supervision. Mentors listened, supported, enabled, and advised, whilst supervisors were authoritarian, overseeing and assessing one's work – and, for the few respondents familiar with supervision in the helping professions, came the view that supervision had the perceived stigmatization of 'personal therapy'.

Mentoring, on the other hand was declared 'user friendly', lacking any implied stigma of either therapy, or authority. To my mind, it had a further advantage in that no doctor appeared to know very much about what mentoring was. It, therefore, had the capacity to become – providing that it worked within a clearly defined mentor-framework and it could retain a more flexible image – an adaptable intervention, which balanced support and nurture with professional challenge and development.

Survey of existing mentor schemes

The second study consisted of a series of unstructured interviews with the co-ordinators of five mentoring projects then in existence in general practice, to ask about their experience of running the scheme, and the objective purpose of their mentoring. The interview was used to ask about the stated objectives of their mentor scheme, and the experience of setting it up and running it. These professional exchanges were very valuable, providing as they did the opportunity to learn from those who have gone before. A recurring theme, significant in these interviews, very relevant to formulating the holistic model, was a sense of general uneasiness amongst mentors when confronted with their mentees' personal feelings. When their mentee had talked of stress at work, of feeling overwhelmed, or disillusioned with general practice their mentor had felt uncomfortable, and freely owned up to their tendency to avoid further discussion, preferring instead to talk of personal learning plans, or career goals. It was clear that these mentors were far from insensitive to the needs of their mentee, but were themselves afraid of entering into what they perceived as being 'dangerous waters' – and here again the dreaded words 'personal therapy' were used.

Such avoidance was related to a further reported difficulty – the lack of clarity in defining their mentor role, a continuing uncertainty which was referred to by all those doctors interviewed. The co-ordinators of these mentor projects had, with their colleagues, decided that a clearer definition of the mentor role would come naturally, from performing it – an understandably pragmatic approach. But this had not resulted in any increase in confidence. Rather than becoming clearer about their task, they became more confused, and consequently less responsive to their mentee's agenda. As if that were not enough, these pioneering mentors reported that they had vastly underestimated the amount of time required to act as mentor, and underestimated the effect that taking on the role would have on themselves. This resulted in their sense of isolation, at times feeling burdened by the material brought to them by their mentee. Despite all of this, their certainty that mentoring was a positive intervention, which brought benefit to their mentee and challenged their own professional learning, was unshaken.

These discussions significantly influenced the structures for delivering the holistic model, and brought a confirmation of the relevance of my previous knowledge and experience. Working within a therapeutic discipline brings a heightened awareness of the need to support those who, in turn, offer support to others, particularly when the support the practitioner gives touches the inner life of others, as it does in the doctor–patient relationship. It also shows the harm that can result from trivializing, or side stepping the personal concerns of others when these have been courageously disclosed, even though such avoidance derives from self protection.

The varying nature of activities described as mentoring in the interviews served not only to heighten confusion about the role and function of a mentor, but undermined the mentor's confidence. This again highlighted the importance of working with a clear definition of the mentor's role and purpose. One negative consequence of this confusion and uncertainty was that the needs of the mentee became eclipsed by the mentor's need to direct the content of the work, keeping it within their reach, rather than allowing for the mentee to set the agenda for discussion and action. Holistic mentoring emphasized the need to make overt the mentee's control of the intervention, giving them ownership of its direction. This in turn required a mentor development programme which encouraged a flexible and open approach to their mentees, one which actively recognized the overlap between personal and professional life, and offered mentors the means by which they could address the preoccupations of their mentee.

These factors also acted to strengthen a personal resolve – to create a model of mentoring that would encourage and sustain mentors to explore with their mentee uncharted seas, rather than sail past them to reach safe, known havens. In this journey of exploration, rather than releasing the chaos they so feared, they might instead discover that the process would yield insights, opportunities for understanding, which would further enhance the personal and professional development of both partners in the relationship. But to achieve this, the work of the mentor had to sit within a clearly defined structure, one which would not constrain their developing skills and knowledge, but which would make the experimentation with their role safe, and ensure that their 'learning-from-doing' was reflected upon, understood within a wider theoretical framework, and rendered useful in consolidating the mentor's knowledge base.

Structure and administration of the mentor scheme

An initial 2 months of concentrated activity was needed to establish structures within which to advertise, deliver, administer and evaluate the product of holistic mentoring, and examples of surrounding documentation which achieved this are included in Chapter 9, which offers a detailed practical guide to getting started. Once a mentor team had been formed, and started work, all these structures would be revised and amended by the mentor team in the light of their experience and feedback from their mentees. This intense activity in fact proved cost effective, for it reduced the time required in the longer term to administer the project.

EVALUATION

The scheme uses an action-research framework. A deceptively simple characterization is that it is an intervention to practice to bring about improvement[4] by active intervention, more fully described in Chapter 7. A significant feature of action research is that evaluation is incorporated into practice, is carried out by practitioners, and is not seen as a separate activity from the project work. To this end, the administrative structures included documentation (which are included in the Appendices) to record the mentor interview, and to be used by the mentor with their mentee as part of their action-planning. The recording sheet also provided some feedback on the major themes of the mentoring session, which, together with an exit questionnaire which seeks anonymous information from mentees on their experience of their mentoring relationship, provided a means whereby the work of the scheme could be monitored, and some feedback given to the mentor team on the process of mentoring. Both the interview-record sheet and the exit questionnaire were developed by the mentor team, in discussion with mentees, so that the balance between confidentiality of the session, and the need to present evidence of its impact on the profession, was comfortably upheld. A software program was developed as a database, which enables the scheme co-ordinator to have a constant overview of mentor workload and availability, number of mentees working within the scheme, number of interviews, etc. – all information which at times is usefully pulled down and presented to those who fund the scheme.

As a general guide to resourcing, the annual budget for a scheme using 20 mentors working with 70 mentees is £25 000–28 000. This allows for a reimbursement to mentors of half-day locum fees, plus travel costs. All meetings associated with mentoring receive Postgraduate Education Allowance (PGEA) accreditation.

FREQUENCY OF MEETINGS

Mentoring relationships are distinguished by their consistency, but the real constraints of mentor time and money had to be balanced against likely demand. The mentors were at one in thinking that it would be for their mentee to determine the frequency of contact, supported by evidence which suggested that, once the initial contact was made and the agenda aired, longer gaps could be managed between sessions. A minimum of three meetings per year was set as the baseline for the activity to qualify as mentoring, with an expectation that they would not exceed five, but this was left entirely to the mentor's discretion – if he or she perceived their mentee to need more than five, then this was accepted. In practice, the average number of meetings per year is five.

ALLOCATION OF MENTEES TO MENTORS

Reflecting further on the literature, and on the experience of those colleagues in other mentor schemes, provided no easy answer to the vexed question of how mentors would be paired with mentees. In schemes which had adopted a policy of 'free choice', circulating information about available mentors and asking the mentee to choose the person most likely to meet their needs, this had resulted in two or three mentors being bombarded with requests, whilst others, inevitably feeling spurned and rejected, were not sought.

The formal nature of the scheme made it unrealistic for either the mentor or mentee to have total freedom of choice about each other, and the decision was made to allocate mentees to mentors primarily from a neutral 'no previous knowledge' basis. This was not easy, as general practice is somewhat incestuous by nature, and the pairing had to be realistically balanced with geographical distance. However, from the start it was made clear to mentees that, if for any reason they were unhappy with their allocated mentor, they could request a re-allocation, without having to provide reasons.

It was in keeping with holistic mentoring to see the pairing as voluntary – in the sense that the mentee themselves decided whether to seek a
mentoring relationship – but formal in the sense that they were allocated a
mentor.

APPOINTMENT OF A MENTOR SCHEME CO-ORDINATOR

In setting up the administrative framework for the project, an unexpected
but crucial feature emerged in the role played by the part-time Project Co-
ordinator, appointed to work for 10 hours a week. In addition to straightforward administration, she had the delicate task of allocating mentors to
mentees. In carrying out this task, the co-ordinator found herself in an
exposed and crucially pivotal position for the project as a whole, as well
as to the individuals within it. The relationship she established with the
mentor team was likened to that of being a lightning conductor – absorb-
ing dynamics of the project, listening patiently over the phone to the
mentors' worries, acting as a sounding board to new ideas, and repeating
information to those who had forgotten, mislaid, or destroyed relevant
documentation. In so doing, she acquired her own perceptions of the
various strengths and weaknesses of the project, and her input into its
development was invaluable, so that she became an unexpected protago-
nist in the new scenario of mentoring. A further consideration in getting
the concept of mentoring established and accepted then has been that
the administrator has the necessary skills, and personality, to go beyond
routine administration, and act as a bridge between the various parties
concerned. To this end, the co-ordinator works closely with the mentor
scheme leader, and plays an active part in attending plenary support meetings, conferences, and seminars, thus maintaining a continuing dialogue
with mentors and leader as the scheme develops.

RECRUITING MENTORS AND THEIR MENTEES

The constraints of the budget, and other resources indicated a targeted
approach to the first trawl for mentors. To this end, the region's 12 GP
tutors were used as the front-runners in advertising for a sales team to
peddle a holistic concept of mentoring. The reason for this was the GP
tutors' more intimate knowledge of their local patch, which was likely to
extend beyond those doctors who turned up for educational events at
their postgraduate centre to an informed overview of the practitioner
scene. First and foremost, the concept of holistic mentoring, and its
rationale had to be sold to the tutors – they themselves had to be convinced of the product's likely worth. To correct the common view of mentoring as being the province of trainers and educators, the importance of
recruiting mentors from the 'rank and file' of general practitioners was
stressed, ensuring that the mentor team represented all walks of the profession. Using primarily a personal approach, backed up with reference to
the scheme in their postgraduate centre meetings, GP tutors promoted the
call for mentors, following through expressions of interest by distributing a
prepared information pack for intending mentors. This contained informa-

tion about the aims and objectives of mentoring, together with the dates of introductory workshops.

As the scheme developed, it advertised itself – informally by word-of-mouth, including recommendations of those being mentored, and formally, through publication, and conference presentations, thus widening the field of potential interest.

Mentees were recruited to the scheme simultaneously, but by different means. In order to avoid swamping newly appointed mentors with an unmanageable demand, and risking discrediting the scheme by keeping mentees waiting months before a mentor became available, geographical parts of the region were addressed in turn. Each doctor in that area was sent a personal letter telling them of the scheme, and enclosing information about the scheme's objectives, and the role and function of a mentor. The entirely voluntary and confidential nature of the mentor–mentee relationship was stressed. Wider advertising came from posters and information sheets distributed in postgraduate centre GP meetings, and eye-catching posters displayed in any place deemed likely to be used by general practitioners. The first trawl of mentees, carried out at the start of the scheme, included practitioners early on in their careers, women doctors balancing career demands with child care, and established practitioners, well settled into professional life, some approaching retirement. This is a continuing spectrum, which provides for the development of an initial database for the scheme, from which to discover more about the effectiveness, or otherwise, of mentoring.

SUPPORT FOR MENTORS

As the previous chapter shows, when mentoring is effective, secondary benefits accrue to the mentor, as well as to their mentee in that their own professional development is enhanced by their mentoring activity. What the literature failed to demonstrate was the criteria by which that benefit could be achieved. Furthermore, from the secondary studies came the importance of preventing the mentors becoming overwhelmed by their task, and carrying their mentees' agendas. The support structures for the mentor team were carefully designed to reflect the same holistic concept being applied to their mentees, namely to support the mentors in their task, develop their learning and understanding, and maximize their own opportunity for professional development.

Two tiers of training and support structures were set up to fulfil these criteria. As a first tier, an induction phase – a series of introductory workshops – offered intending mentors a definition of task, a knowledge base, identification and initial rehearsal of basic mentor skills, and an introduction to the Reflective Cycle as a further mentoring tool. The second tier, known as mentor support groups, provides the mentors with consistent, ongoing support for their work, addressing their own learning agendas as mentors, and seeking to extend and develop skills, knowledge and understanding of their task, and its relationship to the wider profession. These mentor support groups have three elements:

Locally based, 6-weekly meetings of mentors in a local patch. These offer immediate and easy access to peer-mentors for support and discussion, through the medium of reflective practice.

Three-monthly workshops. These meetings bring the entire mentor team together, in which the whole team comes together to address the development of the scheme, share ideas for review and amendment of procedures, and work with an external resource (usually from outside of medicine) to facilitate further learning.

Developmental days, held three times per year. These are educational days which take learning themes previously drawn up by mentors in their workshop, and offer input designed to extend knowledge and skills in areas relevant to mentoring.

This second, supportive tier has emerged as a critical element in establishing and developing the scheme. Both tiers – initial training and ongoing support – had to be realistically matched to the constraints of general practice, otherwise maintaining and developing one's mentor role would be seen not as a challenging opportunity for individual professional development, but as a further demand on an already overloaded work schedule.

DESIGNING THE INTRODUCTORY WORKSHOPS – FURTHER CONSIDERATIONS

Having set up a framework for the scheme, and with a potential mentor team gathering in the wings, came the somewhat awesome realization that ideas were about to become reality.

The stated aim of the introductory workshops was to enable mentors to work freely and confidently at their task, maximizing potential for their own professional development. The overall objectives were defined as building a supportive framework for the regional mentor team, from which to identify and explore themes relevant to the development of mentoring in general practice, and extend the knowledge base.

The workshops began with participants defining their own concept of mentoring, before comparing these with those used by other professions. Then came the tricky bit, where the holistic model, and its relevance to general practice was introduced and discussed. This was followed by an identification of basic mentor skills, which were rehearsed through the introduction of the Reflective Cycle – a strategy designed to get mentoring off to a purposeful start, and advertise its difference from other forms of helping interventions. The workshops used an interactive teaching style, not simply because this was appropriate to the event, but to allow for the individual attitude of each participant towards becoming a mentor to show through, to have free expression.

In contemplating the design of the all-important introductory workshops, and emerging from the planning which preceded their construction, came four considerations: structure, style, selection, and scene setting.

The structure of the introductory workshop again recognized the inherent difficulty of recruiting from a demoralized and overloaded workforce. Capturing the interest of busy practitioners, and encouraging them to attend the introductory workshop, was only half the battle. If the learning required for the task was perceived as overwhelming, and unfamiliar, it would reduce any further motivation for doing it. The workshop had to construct new learning for mentoring which from the outset appeared manageable to participants.

Related to this was the teaching style adopted in the delivery of the workshops. A previous chapter addressed the preference of general practitioners for largely self-directed learning, yet the secondary studies undertaken also showed that general practitioners had no broad knowledge or understanding of mentoring as a concept. The teaching needed to carefully balance an inductive, learner-centred approach with an information giving, didactic element.

The workshops were also the first testing ground for the accuracy and relevance of the holistic model, when the participant's response to the ideas would show whether they appeared relevant, sensible, and manageable. To that end, presenting the rationale behind the model required clarity and coherence, balanced with a sufficiently open teaching style which encouraged verbalized disagreement, and was flexible enough to allow for amendments to the model to be incorporated into the model as the learning process progressed.

In this way, the workshops were openly declared as a two-way learning process – for the workshop leader as well as participants. They were also seen as a two-way selection process. Potential mentors could find out more about mentoring and the holistic model, and consider their future involvement, whether they wanted to work with myself as their leader. At the same time, each individual's responses and interaction in the group would provide me with some evidence as to whether he or she already possessed, or could quickly develop, the flexibility, openness, and sensitivity appropriate to the task. Those members who seemed not to possess the right qualities had to be dissuaded, without causing offence.

Beyond this were the wider considerations of how to help mentors get started. I saw the initial mentoring interview as a considerable challenge, setting the scene for what was to follow.

The conversations in the secondary studies referred to earlier, and my own previous knowledge and experience, showed how crucial was the first meeting between mentor and mentee to the establishment of a professional relationship. Leff[5] is quite brutal in telling all those embarking on a helping relationship that, if you don't 'get it right' in the first 20 minutes, you might as well pack up and go home – a somewhat sweeping statement perhaps, but one which infers how the opening interview demonstrates to the mentee (or otherwise) the trustworthiness of their mentor, and their confidence in their task. Yet, cruelly, this is the time the mentor would feel most vulnerable, feeling, quite rightly, that they were being assessed, and therefore anxious to 'get it right'.

What strategy could be devised which would sustain new mentors to establish a professional discussion, and together with their mentee build a purposeful working agenda, rather than slip into the anecdotal conversation I feared would be born from initial uncertainty and lack of confidence? If the initial scene was set by the latter, not only would it be harder for both mentor and mentee to move out of it at a later stage, but mentoring would be perceived as a friendly chat rather than a professional exchange, and immediately lose credibility. More important, its distinction as a developmental, supportive, yet focused and purposeful relationship would be obscured. These were the factors that underpinned the development of the Reflective Cycle.

Part 2: The reflective cycle

Mentoring, like other developmental interviewing, moves through three stages:

Establishing phase (beginning the mentoring relationship)
Ongoing phase (the middle of the relationship)
Ending phase (closing the relationship, ending and summarizing the work)

The Reflective Cycle was a strategy designed to help the mentor and their mentee overcome the potential hurdles previously described in the establishing phase.[6] An additional aim was to provide for the mentee an introduction to the nature of professional mentoring, and emphasize the holistic, developmental aspects of the relationship.

However, for the mentors it had to be a strategy that announced itself fairly quickly as an aid to their work, not an encumbrance. It needed to be familiar to potential mentors, half-recognized or 'known' so that they felt confident about using it. The Kolb learning cycle[7] (Figure 3.1) is familiar, frequently referred to in continuing education:

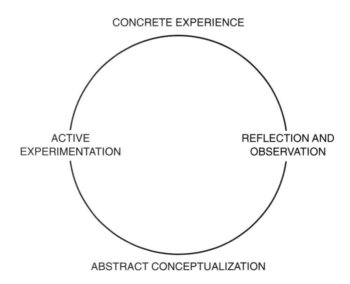

Figure 3.1 Kolb learning cycle

By moving around the stages in a cycle – from concrete experience, to reflection and analysis of the experience, into identifying conceptual frameworks which inform the experience, and finally application of these by active experimentation – new learning is integrated from which knowledge, skills and attitudes consolidate, develop, and are refined over time. Failure to complete the cycle leads to partial or total loss of learning opportunities.

The Reflective Cycle replaced the Kolb learning cycle with one which moved around the various components of personal and professional life, exploring each component to identify hindrances, locate strengths, and find opportunities for achieving a positive future. Like the Kolb model, the cycle upheld the importance of reflection on experience, and reinforced the developmental concept of mentoring as one which moved through stages. It also introduced mentors to three concepts important to effective mentoring, which, through their ongoing support groups could be revisited, and re-encountered through their experience of mentoring.

The first concept was to recognize the relationship between personal and professional life. Griffiths and Tann,[8] seeing the divide between theory and practice as false, argue that the public, external theory of a profession is translated into practice through the medium of the practitioners' personal theories, which in turn stem from their own personal values. Central to the spirit of reflective practice, they say, is reflection on the personal and professional concerns of the practitioner.

The Reflective Cycle, together with a set of open-ended introductory questions, was envisaged as a tool for facilitating reflection on these concerns, with the mentor helping the mentee to see how their personal theories influenced their professional practice; the inclusion of questions about original motivation to become a general practitioner were designed to encourage this reflection. It moved the holistic model firmly towards Carruthers' second category of mentoring,[9] where the mentor addresses both personal and professional issues, and implies that the mentor is flexible, capable of working in both areas.

The second concept was to understand life experience as a series of transitional stages. Developmental psychology offers models of self-development in which the personality develops through stages from infancy to old age, and these were significant in Levinson *et al.*'s[10] earlier work on male mentoring relationships. Like Levinson *et al.*, the work of the mentoring team continues to be strongly influenced by Erikson's[11] concept of identity and the life cycle. At different stages in life, various psycho-social tasks appear, which, if the personality is to grow and develop, have to be confronted and worked through. Encountering these, we reflect on our experience of them, sometimes discussing them with significant others. This reflective process helps the acquisition of new knowledge and skills in resolving the dilemmas which life poses. Moving in this way through the stages and events of our life, we accumulate knowledge and confidence, enabling us to maximize our potential as stable and fulfilled adults.

It seemed more than likely that those who sought out a mentor would themselves be confronting one of life's dilemmas – entering general practice, attempting to survive it, or considering exiting from it. By using the

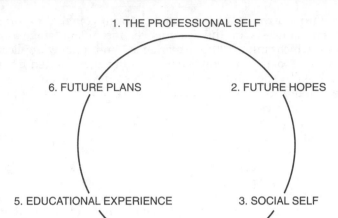

Figure 3.2 The Reflective Cycle

Reflective Cycle (Figure 3.2), mentors could actively explore both concepts, and be introduced to a third, central concept of holistic mentoring which is to view dilemmas not necessarily as 'problems' but as transitions. Transitions move us on, from one stage to another, having all the potential of a positive outcome. From this perspective, confronting problems and apparent obstacles to life did not necessarily risk danger, or chaos, but could be viewed instead as opportunities to gain insight, and identify undiscovered strengths. Once in this position, the mentor could more positively help their mentee re-order and recreate their world.

To each part of the Reflective Cycle was attached an introductory set of open-ended questions. These would be rehearsed in the introductory workshop, and offer a model of exploratory interviewing, which would go beyond superficial exchanges, and would define some essential mentor skills, such as open-ended questioning, and listening with genuine attention. The questions were suggestions, which could be reviewed and amended as mentors developed their style of work.

The questions devised were as follows:

1. The professional self

Why general practice?

Tell me about your role in the practice – what role do you see yourself undertaking?

What role do you enjoy most?

What do you feel about general practice now?

Can you describe the most difficult incident/event in the practice in the last 6 months?

What was your response?

How do you think your partners and staff view you?

In putting the 'professional self' at the start of the cycle, and in formulating these questions, I was hoping to begin with the 'safe' area of professional identity. The first three questions might encourage reflection on what motivating factors, or incidents in life, brought the mentee into general practice, so that they could begin to chart their professional journey, and share something of their work context and role with their mentor. This safe start might be followed by some more searching questions about possible professional disenchantment, or aspects of work that were difficult. The catalytic questions about how they might be perceived by others in their professional role encouraged reflection from which to develop further insight.

2. Future hopes

Where do you want to be in 5 years' time?
Are you on course for achieving this?
What do you identify as your personal strengths?
Can we identify which forces will hinder your future plans?
Which forces will act positively on future plans?
What do you see as your greatest achievement?

These questions built on the 'safe start' by encouraging the mentee to reflect on their future career. It would identify those who were reactive to professional life, and were simply washed along on the tide of events, and those who had a goal plan, a vision for their future, and had at least begun the process of identifying what they needed to be doing in order to achieve it. Identifying hindering and helping forces to their career progression should also feed the construction of a working agenda for the mentoring relationship; asking about achievements balanced the exploration of negative forces with the positive strengths which the mentee possessed for overcoming them.

3. Social self

How do you spend your time when you are not working?
How would your best friend describe you?
What do you gain from your social interests and activities?
Do you feel you actively make time for outside interests – or simply use what time is left over after work commitments are fulfilled?
What do you look for in your relationships with friends?

Here the more personal aspect of self was introduced, to consider professional life alongside personal life. As with the previous questions, it would help the mentors ascertain how far the mentees were in control of their lives, whether they were simply surviving work, or (more concerning) whether social life was receding in the face of work demands. The questions also continued the theme of insight into self – how aware the mentees were of their own needs in relationships, and their effect on others.

4. Personal self

Tell me about the people who most influenced your formative years.
What characterizes your own upbringing?
What sort of person would you describe yourself as being?
What events/circumstances do you find most stressful?
To whom do you turn for support?
To whom do you offer support?

These questions most obviously entered the personal arena. Again, I had in mind the element of self-awareness, the knowledge of self, and responses to events and critical incidents. I was thinking also about the influences of early life on career choice, and awareness of significant people and events.

5. Educational experience

What has been your most enjoyable educational experience?
Why was it enjoyable?
Can you give me an example of a negative learning event?
What effect might this have had on you?
What is your preferred style of learning?
What are (a) your strengths in learning and (b) your limitations in learning?
In what areas would you like to increase skills and knowledge?

Questions like these moved the mentoring focus back onto safer, more familiar ground after excursions into (perhaps) less comfortable areas. Again, I thought that previous learning history would be important to explore, as it might affect present learning patterns, and indeed the mentoring relationship itself, and links could be made between this and earlier questions about future hopes.

6. Future plans

Define three objectives for your professional development.
Can we clarify learning needs related to these objectives?
What would you see as being obstacles to your professional development?
What would you see as our future working agenda?
Are there other areas of discussion you would like to develop, or return to?

In many ways, the Reflective Cycle is a route map – an aid to begin a journey, something to be discarded once the journey begins, and more useful or interesting ways of getting to a goal have been discovered. The decision as to whether to use the map was then, as it is now, entirely the mentor's. Some mentees come to their mentor with a clear idea of what is on their agenda, and plunge straightaway into the process of working through it, needing no help in establishing the work. But, for others less certain, the Reflective Cycle was intended to help the mentee, as well as their mentor in the difficult business of getting started. In the early interviews, the mentor would take their mentee around the cycle, inviting them to recall the experience relevant to that stage, reflect upon it, and use it as an exploratory base from which to identify factors which were currently promoting or hindering their professional wellbeing.

In the mentee's experience of being carefully listened to, as they responded to the questions attached to the cycle, might come active encouragement for purposeful reflection, to 'hear their own voice'. The major decisions in life are often taken intuitively; having taken them, we seldom revisit the scene to look again at the circumstances that brought the decision about. Yet understanding the process by which we arrived at where we are now is an essential component to moving on, and forward – the transitional stage. The attention and interest of the mentors in their mentees' answers to the questions could aid the process of constructing their own map, and help formulate their life plans more clearly.

Finally, questions which might shape the formation of a plan for the future, and identify ways in which the objectives of the plan could be achieved, formed an important end-stage. Identifying obstacles to professional development was one of the declared tasks of the holistic mentor, one essential to address from early on in the relationship, so that the mentee felt the acknowledgement that comes from being heard and understood.

So, we had undertaken the reflective analysis, formulated some abstract concepts, and next was the acid test of experimentation – the concrete experience that would either declare the Reflective Cycle as another good idea that bit the dust, or a strategy that had potential. To this end, the Reflective Cycle was rehearsed in the introductory workshops. Working in pairs gave participants a taste of what it was like to be both on the receiving end of searching, open-ended questions, and being responsible for asking them sensitively. One partner would choose one of the six phases of the cycle, deciding in which area they wanted to work. Their partner then asked them the developmental questions attached to that stage, before changing over, to ensure that both participants had the experience of being both a mentor and a mentee.

This workshop experience was intended to act as a practical demonstration of the supportive, yet challenging and purposeful nature of holistic mentoring. The concepts which underpin the Reflective Cycle were revisited during the second, following tier of training and support; and the strategy, like everything else in the scheme, was amended, and developed through use. But that leaps ahead of the story – firstly, how did the potential mentors receive their introduction to this and other aspects of the mentoring task?

Part 3: Experience of the introductory workshops

Eight introductory workshops were held over a period of 6 months, and all provided a rich source of feedback on participants' response to the holistic model, and the Reflective Cycle. In all of the workshops, participants were established general practitioners, aged (approximately) 40–45 years, with approximately one third of the participants being women. Overall, the majority of participants were in practice partnerships, although in one workshop the work context of the participants meant that 10 out of 14 participants were in single-handed practice. Whilst the interest of a very few participants was prompted by requests from their regional adviser, the majority of the participants were self selected and voluntary.

The described experience of the introductory workshop focuses on two areas:

● The participants' perceived definition of mentors and their reaction to the holistic model
● Their experience of using the Reflective Cycle.

Defining mentoring

All the workshops opened with participants discussing their own definitions and concepts of a mentor's role and function. Some of these are included here, for they provide an interesting snapshot of how general practitioners view mentor roles, and will be a useful starting point for those readers implementing their own mentor schemes. In the workshops, these definitions were put alongside those emerging from the literature, and the models of mentoring used in other professions. In this way, differences and similarities could be declared, and those members with individual agendas, or fixed ideas about the task, could have space to say where they were coming from in their interpretation of the word.

Most, but not all of the participants saw mentors as someone who listened, who facilitated the 'looking at self', offering insight and support. One group included 'equipping people for change', alongside giving advice, and offering different perspectives on problems. 'Enabling facilitator' seemed to sum up the dominant view, although on closer inspection, more precise definitions of 'facilitation' showed less certain understandings of that concept.

Naturally, each of the workshop groups took on a particular identity, and undoubtedly this influenced their definition of the task. For example, one group contained three doctors who had attended additional training in counselling, holistic medicine, and alternative therapies. They were articulate and energetic, taking others along with them in their obvious enthusiasm for the potential task, but this created two problems. Firstly, they tended to see mentoring as an extension of their counselling role, allowing them access to doctors with identified 'problems', and they needed consistent reminding that mentoring was not personal therapy. Secondly, their enthusiasm made it difficult at times to hear clearly, and without interruption, the voices of those who were cautious about becoming an enabler, but sought instead a more defined role as 'trusted teacher' or 'professional guide'.

In another group, the climate was suspicious, and at times hostile, infected by the obvious depression of one member, and the obvious disapproval of another; so that maintaining a reasonably positive climate in which the other group members could work was a constant struggle. In contrast, a third group contained some vociferous 'brand leaders' in general practice, and here the struggle was to contain the discussion, and keep to its focus, as all participants entered into this workshop with great energy and engagement.

As the opening sessions unfolded, discussion in the various groups gave further evidence of the motivating factors for people's interest in exploring the mentor role in general practice. Various statements were made:

'I feel so much the loss of collegiality in our profession'

and many participants referred to the changed, current professional climate:

'we need to replace competition with co-operation – to re-instate sharing and support'

and commented that whilst fundholding had served to integrate practice groups, through the new and necessary shared element of the task, a (regrettable) element of competitiveness had crept in.

There were also some interesting polarizations. In one group, the definitions of a mentor were exclusively focused on the educational, teaching role of the mentor, as someone who would 'oversee continuing education plans', 'offer support for learning', 'help people prepare for the MRCGP exams'. Tentative suggestions that mentors might also be catalysts for change were met with palpable anxiety – this would 'open up cans of worms', and, guess what, lead to 'personal therapy'. For this group, educational supervision was the overriding definition, for it was considered 'dangerous' to consider anything other than this clearly identified task.

In all groups, the enthusiasm and confidence displayed in defining the mentor's role was tempered with anxiety. This anxiety was located in the notion that mentors might also have to be 'all wise and all knowing' and 'have stature, greater knowledge, obvious standing' – the wise father of Homeric mentoring.

In sharp contrast, the element of wisdom, did not, however, worry one group. They collectively defined mentors as 'wise', as 'gurus', as 'masters', 'masters of excellence, from whom others can learn'. One member said enthusiastically:

'they [mentees]will sit at my feet and learn from me how all things are done – I will tell them how it is so'.

These guru-mentors were also given additional responsibilities as 'advice-givers' and 'problem solvers'. All the participants in this group were from an Eastern culture, and rightly perceived the role of a mentor from within that cultural tradition, where mentors are masters, and gurus. Whilst initially their definition appeared far removed from those of their peers in other geographical groups, and from those described in the literature, it was an important first lesson in learning to work *within* their understanding, starting from where they were, rather than where I, as the group facilitator, thought they should be. As Chapter 8 shows, these mentors introduced me to a personal learning curve on the importance of culture, and I am indebted to them for their patience with me.

Overall, although the teaching style in the workshops encouraged disclosure, openly stating that all contributions were valuable when working with an unknown phenomenon, some members nevertheless remained wary of disclosing their thoughts about the mentor role. For some, still nursing the scars of their medical training and unfamiliar with working in small groups, the somewhat exposed, open style of the workshop was difficult. They would have preferred, I am sure, a safer, less engaged position in the learning process but, when encouraged, their responses often accelerated the discussion, for example:

'mentoring goes beyond befriending – it is much more complex than that'

and

'there must be something that makes it work – we need to get into identifying and understanding the factors that make it happen'.

Would holistic mentoring be a model that made 'it' happen?

Introducing holistic mentoring

In almost all of the groups, introducing participants to the holistic model of mentoring, with its three components of education, personal support and professional development, brought an unexpected air of excitement, not a response normally associated with groups of doctors. It seemed that the holistic model made sense to practitioners, suggesting that the assessment of need on which it was based was accurate, which is always good news to educationalists. But more importantly it shifted participants away from what they thought mentoring *might* be to what they saw it could *become*. Excitement accompanied the growing realization that, provided they had a flexible framework which was linked to other professional mentor models, they could be the ones who, by their work with mentees, began to define and create the mentor model for their own profession – as pioneers and protagonists. These participants sniffed the scent of organizational change.

But in the group that favoured education as the sole focus of mentoring, participants were overwhelmed not by excitement, but anxiety. This stemmed from the idea of mentors offering personal support:

'you need to think what you are doing here – opening cans of worms, and the like'

whilst another participant felt it too closely resembled

'a confessional – with the mentor as priest'

and this tide of anxiety overwhelmed the entire group when one of their members, who had a hierarchical role, declared:

'this is far too dangerous – who knows what we could be getting ourselves into here'.

Delivered as something of an edict, this moved the group back into discussion of the requisite skills required to help mentees build learning portfolios, and devise learning plans; when these were produced the group visibly relaxed. Once the model moved back into the tighter framework of education, leaving aside the other two components, it became acceptable, but it was clear that this intended activity owed little to mentoring, and much more to educational support.

Later reflections on possible reasons for this very different response were illuminating, and gave prominence to the *political expedience* of mentoring, referred to by Morle,[12] and nicely depicted in recent Government moves to shift resources for teacher-training out of universities and into schools. In this case, the student-teacher is assigned a 'mentor' who in effect bears almost total responsibility for the development of their student's knowledge and competence – a role unpopular with teaching staff because of its unreasonable demands, but popular with the head teacher because it brings in additional resources to the school, making it politically expedient to have on hand some willing mentors. For this workshop group, which worked in an area where overcoming the difficulty of promoting continuing education in a scattered, rural community was high on the local political agenda, mentors were seen in part as the potential agents of this policy.

In another group, the political powers saw mentoring as a vehicle from which to address concerns about *cultural* issues, seeing that mentoring might assist the many West Indian and Asian doctors in their region to come up to the professional standards of their white peers – *competence disguised as culture*. The task of mentors was seen as one which could address competence through monitoring performance, and offer an avenue to quality control. This did not sit at all easily with the voluntary, supportive nature of holistic mentoring, creating a potential division between what the organization saw as the benefits of mentoring, and what potential mentors themselves perceived the benefits to be.

These two factors highlighted an important omission in the thinking behind the original formulation of the holistic model. Mindful of the organizational and professional context in which the model might sit, considerably less thought had been given to the *local* context of mentoring. But these local issues could serve to divide the paymasters from the troops – and, as paymasters are providers of funding for mentor schemes, this split in objectives meant that some potential mentors doubted the viability of the model, not because the model itself was flawed (although it could turn out to be so) but because they doubted that it was an appropriate strategy given local, political agendas.

A second workshop group also experienced anxiety rather than excitement at the thought of practising holistic mentoring, but their anxiety centred on boundaries. Drawing clear boundaries to the mentor's task, and keeping within them was an issue for all groups, and rightly so, as they are essential to effective mentoring. The other groups accepted my view that being clear about what you were aiming to do as a mentor, and recognizing where mentoring ended and other types of interventions began did, in itself, help to prevent the Pandora-like chaos some mentors feared would occur if they explored the preoccupations of their mentee. Most participants at least were prepared to go along with this concept, investing some trust in my personal and professional authority as leader, and recognizing that the following support groups would give help and support if they felt troubled. However, where anxiety was the dominant theme, my professional belief, based on conceptual knowledge and experience, proved an insufficient base from which to persuade participants to test it out for themselves. It was stalemate it seemed, for I *'had no language with which to comment on our true predicament . . . whilst they could but experience it inarticulately, through our symptoms and our dread'*[13] (p. 32).

In one of these groups, the dread *was* articulated, via a series of imagined scenarios which, with increasing awfulness, depicted mentors working with the deranged, the drug addicted, the suicidal mentee, leaving the mentor wrung out, overwhelmed by disaster and irresolvable problems. There was an encouraging difference, however, for in this group their anxiety decreased when distinctions were drawn between crisis intervention and mentoring, and was further dispelled when linking the possibility of encountering difficult material in mentoring with being in receipt of information about a 'sick doctor'. In the same way that a sick colleague would be referred to an appropriate specialist who was better able to address an entrenched major problem, the occasional crisis encountered through mentoring could also be referred on. Furthermore, there was an overall acceptance that, realistically, mentoring would be unlikely to appeal to those who were 'sick', in the same way that the depressed, or deeply stressed patient is unable to actively seek help.

In this second group, anxiety focused on 'knowing' the distinction between counselling and mentoring. One participant asked:

'as mentors, are we being fake counsellors – given a licence to practise simply by being a GP?'

There is a clear distinction between interpreting unconscious behaviour and intent, as part of a counselling relationship where the *counsellor* is charged with actively *doing* something with what they have heard, against the mentor's more passive role of acknowledging that they have heard, and encouraging the *mentee* to explore it. But within this discussion was an interesting contradiction. In my educational work with doctors, it has not been uncommon for me to be told that counselling is part and parcel of the GP's job – something which every doctor does for a significant part of their time. An absence of training in relevant skills is not generally considered an impediment. Yet, when faced with the possibility of employing similar basic skills with their peers, potential mentors adopted a different stance, in which any such knowledge was denied. The answer to this puzzle emerged later, when the mentors brought back their experiences of mentoring to the support groups.

Overall, the majority of participants in all of the workshops had, by the end of the morning sessions, demonstrated an increasing interest in working at the mentor task, and levels of energy and engagement in the learning process were high. A second paradigm shift took place here, which moved the focus of group discussions past the *why* of mentoring, onwards to the *how* – a promising move – but the real test was yet to come, for, if doctors accepted intellectually the need for a mentoring structure, yet felt unable to carry it out by becoming mentors themselves, the concept could not be fully implemented.

The Reflective Cycle – participants' responses

Accordingly, the Reflective Cycle was introduced carefully, with explanations of the two main themes underpinning it. All groups accepted unquestioningly that the initial meeting between the mentor and their mentee would be crucial in establishing their professional relationship, seeing some parallel between this and meeting a new patient. They were also in accord with a view of mentoring that declared at the outset its purposeful, developmental nature, its difference from a social exchange, although they were concerned that this should not imply any loss of friendliness.

Explaining that the Reflective Cycle was designed to reflect this sense of purpose, and bridge the vulnerable gap between the introductory stage of checking each other out and more focused work, the pairs were set up for their first rehearsal of it in practice. One partner asked developmental questions in the area of the other's choice, using the set questions, or devising their own. Each pair had private space within which to work, allaying concerns about eavesdropping, and reminding participants of the practical structures to ensure confidentiality. Deliberately, requisite skills in interviewing were not identified at this point, but delayed until participants had experience from their use of the Reflective cycle to which to refer.

The dominant theme emerging from their collective experience of using the Reflective Cycle was the participant's feeling of being challenged. As doctors are most often in the role of asking questions and taking control, being on the receiving end of open-ended questions was for many a new experience. Further responses to the experience fell into two categories: a *personal* response to the experience of being 'developmentally questioned' and a *professional* 'mentor' response to the implications of using the model in practice.

For the majority, the personal experience of responding to the developmental questions illustrated the potential power in the (comparatively) simple process of being allowed an opportunity to reflect on experience, and explore the outcomes with a trusted peer. In their feedback, they discovered that:

'we could have talked for hours'

(although not everyone expected to)

'at first I thought what on earth will I talk about . . . in fact I had the opposite problem – trying to stop'.

All groups commented that their enjoyment of their freedom to talk stemmed largely from not being dogged by feelings of guilt or greed at having uninterrupted time for themselves:

'over half an hour . . . just about me'

'when you spend most of your time listening to patients there is a tremendous sense of freedom in being listened to – and carefully listened to . . . by a peer'.

Some participants discovered the re-energizing quality of purposeful reflection:

'I feel differently about the job now, just having talked about it . . . more enthusiastic'

'Talking to P . . . I realized something about my partnership that has never struck me before'.

These rehearsals had a secondary benefit. Sharing experience in this way bonded the groups together, through a sense of shared discovery:

'surprising really – after only a day together I feel I really know people here'

and this was an unforeseen benefit when it came to forming a mentor team, as this previous knowledge was carried forward into establishing a team identity.

Within the category of professional response, the idea of constructing mentor interviews along developmental cycles was quickly grasped, but this experiential learning turned out to be a two-edged sword. On the personal side, group members were taken aback that such a simple and manageable structure could have striking results, and found it useful in formulating their thoughts, and moving the discussion forward. But on the *professional* side was the realization that using the cycle could, as one potential mentor put it:

'take you further faster'

and they felt the power of this acutely, saying

'hey . . . this is hot stuff'

and

'this is a radical departure from the stiff upper lip of our medical training'.

The implications of travelling fast provoked much discussion in this introductory stage, and became a continuing theme in the ongoing support workshops. At the heart of this was empowerment. The rehearsal sessions in these introductory workshops allowed a glimpse of the future, and the potential power of mentoring. The sense of power was intimidating, but was balanced with a growing confidence that a flexible mentoring framework, which had allegiance to other professional models, could make possible the introduction of an in-house support network for general practice. Participants saw how they could become pioneers, defining and creating mentoring for their own profession, and could be heard turning over this possibility in their minds:

'there is a real possibility that this would work . . . we could make it work'

and

'the profession has been looking for this for some time . . . the trouble is we didn't know what "it" was' whilst considering more carefully how they, as individuals, might want to interpret the mentor model:

'I don't know how to say this . . . but simply doing the educational bit would be so boring . . . for them [the mentee] and us'

and

'surely mentoring would be so limiting if it was only about one thing – exploring feels good'.

Exchanges after experiencing the Cycle echoed earlier comments which could be construed as motivating factors:

'we have lost our collegiate feeling for each other – this is a way back, towards supporting each other rather than competing with each other'

With a concrete experience to reflect upon, discussions in all groups swung back into being mindful of the necessity to keep appropriate boundaries for the mentor's task, but now the concerns could be taken up by the membership. For example, one group pondered about how far to go in exploring issues which belonged to personal life yet clearly got in the way of professional life, like having an unsupportive spouse or life partner. Participants could now put forward their own experience of drawing boundaries, as one doctor said:

'well . . . it's hard to describe . . . but you know it when you see it – or rather you sense it, you draw back'

and could more spontaneously draw parallels from experience with patients and friends.

At this point it seemed right that I should stand back, to withdraw from the exploratory learning process. A model of mentoring had been offered, and now the likely purveyors of that model had to use their experience of it to decide its viability or otherwise.

Using the Reflective Cycle prompted some 'road to Damascus' experiences, sources of enjoyable enlightenment. For example, during the morning session, one group found themselves divided into two camps. There were the 'believers' – those on the whole prepared to give the ideas a whirl, and there were the 'doubters' who constantly presented the believers with the obstacles to implementing mentoring. They told them that the impetus for mentoring was not there in the grass roots of their professional community, that doctors would see mentoring as an imposition. In any case, how would they, as busy doctors find the time to become mentors? And another thing, if they did, who would pay for it?

More reluctantly, but obediently, the doubting group agreed to try out the Reflective Cycle exercise, and then, having overrun the allotted time, confidently announced to their stunned colleagues that:

'Mentoring is THE answer – and retired GPs can do it'

and when they did it would 'prevent isolation, and burn-out' and 'help doctors to manage change', 'avoid wastage' and be a 'safety valve' for the mentee . . . the list was endless.

A similar Damascus experience was undergone in another group, who had, at the beginning of the introductory workshop, given themselves the title of the 'Holy Grail' group, for they thought this summed up their joint quest for 'right answer' to a myriad of complex questions prompted by the concept of mentoring. They collectively anticipated that the Reflective Cycle would be an enjoyable activity, entering into it with gusto, after which they all declared:

'the search is ended . . . *everybody* should have one [a mentor]'.

These instant conversions summoned up glorious pictures of hapless doctors cowering in postgraduate centres and surgeries, hiding from evangelical mentors who roamed the region, preaching the deliverance that comes from mentorship, intent on converting practitioners to the new faith of mentoring. But Stephenson[14] goes ahead of such prophets, telling of the danger of seeing the vogue of mentoring as a panacea for all ills, applied in answer to all manner of problems, and she presents instead a thoughtful treatise about the relevant application of mentoring.

Returning to the context of applying this holistic mentoring model to general practice, the experience gained in using the Reflective Cycle once more highlighted the relative isolation of general practitioners, giving testimony to the paucity of time and opportunity for purposeful reflection. A thematic analysis of eight group discussions following the use of the Reflective Cycle, showed clearly that, whilst the focus of the introductory workshops had been to introduce mentoring as a commodity on offer to other practitioners, the purveyors of that commodity wanted some for themselves. My interruption of one pair, half an hour over their allotted time and working steadily through their tea break, was greeted by:

'oh good heavens . . . we cannot stop now . . . my dear lady we have only just begun'.

Their body language suggested that they were deeply engaged, and in all of the groups, it proved extremely difficult to keep the exercise within its time boundaries. This upheld the expensive inclusion of the two-tier support groups within the overall framework of the scheme, for it implied that, before mentors set out to feed and support others, they firstly needed to feed themselves. On the basis of this observation, the dates for the first meetings of the support group were brought forward to ensure that they were convened within 2 weeks of the first mentoring interview.

For the group of Asian mentors, the Reflective Cycle was a means of discovering another dimension of being a guru, and with the benefit of their Eastern perspective, this group quickly recognized and mastered the art of reflection:

'I see now what this thing . . . mentoring . . . is. It is like holding up a mirror . . . I will hold up the mirror, and we will both look into it'.

This activity of shared reflection, so perfectly encapsulated in the previous comment, was a central feature of their discussion, and even in this early stage showed its capacity for bringing new teaching and learning to relevant areas.

Finally, using the Reflective Cycle gave participants a chance to discard a perception of mentors as all-knowing, with wise answers to life's various problems. Their experience of working with each other had provided a glimpse of the catalytic nature of mentoring. In this last group, their reflective experience brought the realization that part of the guru's power was to encourage exploration, voiced in another perfectly expressed phrase:

'after all Buddha did not tell the answers – and this is what we must be doing; we must take them down the path but not tell them where the answer lies'.

Taken overall, it seemed that despite initial doubts, caution, anxieties and occasional hostility about the applicability of mentoring to general practice, a significant majority of participants shared an understanding of the concepts of holistic mentoring, accepted the rationale on which it was based, and actively endorsed the Reflective Cycle as a meaningful, and manageable strategy.

Its use revealed it was a two-edged sword, in that it demonstrated to participants the potential depth of the mentoring relationship, which was both a challenge, and a responsibility. Potential mentors viewed working in this way with both excitement, and awe, and felt keenly the responsibility of working alongside their peers, wanting to do their best for them, and offer them the best of themselves:

'we need to be sure that at the very least we do no harm . . . we need to develop and grow through the experience so that we get it right for our colleagues'.

If they were not to be all wise and knowing omnipotent gods (and goddesses) of the future, how could they ensure that they had at least the basic skills to became effective catalysts? How could such skills be developed within the limited time scale of an introductory workshop?.

Part 4: Requisite skills in mentoring

Three-stage model

Confronting the somewhat awesome responsibility of mentoring work at least opened the window of opportunity for describing how the second, following tier of training would support the mentors' conscious need to extend present skills, and promote their own development.

To put this into context, a three-stage model briefly referred to earlier in this chapter, was outlined. This identifies three phases in a helping relationship: the crucial *establishing* phase, where skills and energy are focused on building the trust and rapport necessary to begin work, the *ongoing* phase, where good communication skills, insight, and problem solving are used to address the tasks identified in the working agenda, and the *end* phase, which calls for skills in reviewing and summarizing the work and outcomes of the mentoring relationship.

These three phases again emphasize the developing nature of a mentoring relationship, and its movement through stages. The continuing training and support for mentors was designed to move in step with the development of the mentoring relationship, using the mentors' developing experience of their role as a learning base. As their relationship with their mentee progressed, they would encounter areas in the work which they needed to know more about, to understand better, or to examine their attitudes towards. In this way, the mentors' learning agenda matched their work, and was met through peer support and learning, opportunistic teaching, and from bringing into the support workshops people from outside medicine with expertise and knowledge relevant to mentoring.

The common postgraduate educational experience of medicine risks superficial learning, brought about through one-off educational events, squeezed into the working day – a pattern almost certainly related to the inherited tension between service commitment and education, when the demands of clinical practice override protected time for reflection and learning. The learner-centred, developing model of mentor education demonstrated that taking on the role of mentor was a commitment to a *continuing* learning process. In the support groups, the mentors gained more than support for their work, for they also addressed their own professional development, ensuring that both they and their mentees maximized their learning opportunities.

In the introductory workshops, such idealism did not appeal to all participants. Some saw mentoring as a much more occasional business, so that the support structure was seen as unnecessarily onerous, demanding more time and accountability than they were prepared to offer. But for the majority of participants, it evidently reassured them that they would not be left to go it alone, and they could see that the introductory workshop was an induction phase, which focused on *basic* skills, sufficient to get mentors into the arena of establishing relationships.

To introduce new learning in a manageable way, basic skills were addressed primarily by identifying those which had similarities with the good consultation. This conveyed the message that the mentor's task did not demand overwhelming amounts of 'new' learning, but was rather a redefinition, a 'honing in' on familiar themes. The three-stage model was used to further identify these as follows:

ESTABLISHING PHASE

Communication skills to establish the relationship:

Paying genuine attention
Listening
    at two levels
    without interruption
    without distortion
Non-verbal communication
Open-ended questioning
Non-judgmental attitudes
Appropriate use of silence.

As the mentoring relationship developed, these skills would become refined through use, and extended to include other models of intervention. They would be carried into the:

ON-GOING PHASE

Where good communication skills would be needed to address these tasks:

Define the mentee's agenda
Identify, then explore relevant areas
Keep boundaries
Monitor the process of the mentoring relationship
Challenge and confront appropriately
Check accuracy – 'this is what I have heard – is this what you said?'

END PHASE

Communication skills to address the tasks of:

Reflecting and analysing where have we been?
Setting future objectives
Summarizing and reviewing the work, and its outcome.

These skills derive from counselling, but are accepted as the basis for a number of activities in which the purpose is to develop the agenda of one person – appraisals, developmental interviews, and the consultation. Whilst they were familiar to practitioners in the context of the consultation, in the workshops we began to unpick their communication skills with patients, reweaving them into the cloth of mentoring, using some well-known concepts of communication.

Models of communication

Balint[15] offered a useful, and familiar model of communication. In his early work at the Tavistock Clinic, he showed how, in the consultation, the drug most frequently used was the doctor himself. The way in which the doctor offers, and uses himself in the doctor–patient relationship influenced the illness process. His groupwork with doctors, begun in the 1950s, created a model for discussing patients which is still in evidence today. Exploring this model encouraged them to see similarities between it and mentoring. How they presented themselves to the mentee, and used the first inter-view, echoed Balint's interest in the *process*. As with the consultation, the way in which they used themselves in mentoring would have the same influence on the outcome.

We also traced the derivation of current professional debates on 'patient-centred medicine' to the Rogerian[16] perspectives on 'person-centred' interventions, where the agenda of the 'client' was prominent. In patient-centred medicine, the doctor took care to keep the consultation centred on where their patient was, avoiding redirecting the patient's thinking to one which fitted the doctor's own agenda; similarly effective mentoring sought a mentee-centred focus. Pitching the level of input to the immediacy of necessary skills, we began to move to identifying the basic skills needed to achieve Balint's self awareness, and Roger's mentee-centredness, making clear that these were first level skills, and teaching on the different models of interventions would come in the second tier of mentor training.

In the introductory workshops, the focal point had been the establishing phase, the skills of paying attention and listening. These were the skills used in the rehearsal of the Reflective Cycle, and were consciously used to move participants into a starting position – if they chose to continue, and become a mentor, more – much more – would come later through the support groups.

Using their reflective experience as an example, we revisited the importance of paying attention by using the three possible attention zones outlined by Burnard:[17]

> *Zone one*, where the counsellor is fully listening to their client and paying attention to all verbal and none verbal clues
>
> *Zone two*, where attention to the client is only partially attended to because the counsellor is pre-occupied with their own thoughts
>
> *Zone three*, where attention is focused, but the counsellor is busy trying to work out his own theories about the client, rather than giving attention:

'he is interpreting what is going on' (p. 110)

We then referred them to Daloz[18] who affirms the essential quality of listening:

'Listening . . . is a powerful intervention, perhaps the most powerful we have as mentors. It is not a passive process, for the good listener is always alert for things of special significance in a tale, and acts, however subtly, on what he hears' (p. 211).

and again used their own experience of being listened to in the Reflective Cycle, and how positive that had been. Listening at two levels meant listening for what was not said, as well as what was said, not interrupting the mentee, but showing through non-verbal cues your attention and interest.

Not distorting what is heard was related back to the 'mentee-centredness' of the holistic model, and contrasted with the more prescriptive style of the consultation.

Concepts about managing problems came from Egan's[19] seminal work, and his first goal of helping:

'the first goal of helping can be stated in terms of the helpers' effectiveness in helping clients move towards more effective problem management. Helpers are effective to the degree that their clients, through client-centred interactions, are in better positions to manage their problem situations and/or develop the unused resources and opportunities to live their lives more effectively' (p. 5).

It was useful to reinforce the concept of 'containing' problems rather than resolving them – problem management and opportunity for development.

Another reinforcement of an earlier message came through emphasizing the purpose of mentoring as a means to professional development, and avoiding the impression that mentoring was for those in crisis, or was always problem centred, on which Egan's model, like other counselling interventions, is based. Daloz[20] reminds us that there is a tendency to assume the passage of change as a painful one, yet for many it is a welcome release from the constraints of a previous life phase. This allowed further opportunities to say that mentoring would be unlikely to attract those overwhelmed by trauma and problems. It would mainly serve those who were either intent on forging ahead, but encountered obstructions or hindrances to their professional development – the hurdles of the transitional journey; or those who sought positive support for already-formed ideas and plans.

This inevitably disappointed those participants in the workshops who had additional counselling training, and perhaps saw mentoring as an opportunity to counsel their colleagues, or were attracted to the idea of themselves in the crisis role. An analogy with general practitioners who join the 'flying doctor' schemes was offered, the 'green light brigade' who rush to motorway accidents with green flashing lights atop their cars. This was an unfortunate choice in one group, where two participants turned out to be founder members of the local flying doctor scheme, but in fact their experience of being at the centre of crisis added a very useful dimension to the discussion, highlighting the distinction between the time-limited nature of crisis intervention, and the longer-term, developing mentoring relationship.

At the end of the workshops, those participants who had selected themselves in, and expressed a continuing interest in becoming a mentor, were given a prepared *Mentor's Handbook*. Included in the handbook was a form to be returned to the co-ordinator, declaring their intention to join, on receipt of which they would be assigned a mentee. A three day 'cooling off' period was suggested before signing up for the job.

In total, the introductory workshops brought together a group of 88 practitioners. In South West Thames, out of 38 doctors came a more than sufficient consensus to implement the holistic model, with a mentor team of 25, three of whom asked to become mentees as well as mentors. Over 3 years, natural wastage, together with the developing experience of knowing what is a manageable number for a mentor team, has resulted in a current team of 20 mentors.

All 16 participants in the workshop held for Asian doctors in another region declared their intention to become mentors – and gurus. In the event, this team has worked alongside the South West Thames team, providing a rich source of shared learning and experience across regional boundaries, some of which is included in later chapters. Occasional contact is maintained with some of the remaining participants from workshops held outside the region, in which it would seem that their experience of the day fired their enthusiasm for formulating and implementing their own models of mentoring, although one group decided later that it was not the right time for them to progress the initiative.

Reviewing learning outcomes

Before delivering the workshops, four themes had been identified which were considered important to their effectiveness, and these are reviewed in the light of the experience.

STRUCTURE AND SETTING THE SCENE

Recruitment to both the introductory workshops, and to the resulting mentor team, was much higher than anticipated, confounding cynics, bystanders, protagonists, and last but not least myself, as project leader. Workshop members held a collective view of the profession's desire for a more co-operative and supportive climate, and they perceived in mentoring a means of achieving it. The structured learning experience of the introductory day conveyed a picture of a role which was relevant, attractive and manageable to many. However, from this came two unexpected features, which together created a paradox in the recruitment and motivation of mentors.

Firstly, using the holistic model showed the potential power of mentoring, the depth of the relationship, and the speed with which that depth could be reached. For many participants, this *heightened* their motivation to do the job, but emphasized their awareness of their responsibility to increase the wellbeing of their peers, so much so that some openly said they would not contemplate doing it without the guarantee of ongoing developmental support. However, for a fewer number of participants, the discovery of mentoring as 'hot stuff' took them beyond their own more constrained view of mentoring as an occasional professional conversation, or a meeting to provide educational support to a peer, and *lowered* their motivation to take on the role.

The second feature was the speed with which participants saw the organizational benefit of mentoring. They saw that they could, by taking on a mentor role, become agents of organizational change. At times they moved closer to being part of that force for change, at other times they stood back, overwhelmed with the significance of being a potential change-agent.

STYLE

On the whole, the style of teaching in the workshops managed the balance between facilitation and telling, instead of assuming a diagnosis, and then offering a prescription, with ongoing treatment. Like the patient, participants preferred a diagnosis, even if later the condition turned out to be something else, and in discussing the treatment plan, it seemed that a more directive stance was welcomed. Nevertheless, I identified strongly with the journeyman in Chapter 2, who sets about his teaching more in order to learn than to teach. Whilst possessing knowledge of relevant theoretical frameworks, and particular models of mentoring, the discussions which centred on the participants' responses to the holistic concept and their use in the Reflective Cycle meant that we were learning alongside each other about the unknown phenomena of mentoring in general practice. This knowing and not-knowing meant that there could be no statement of certainty – 'this will work' – but instead the lesser offering of 'this is likely to work'.

SELECTION

The introductory workshops introduced the challenge of selecting mentors. Was this challenge met? I doubt it. Darling[21] coined the wonderful phrase 'toxic mentors', providing a gallery of toxic types gathered from experiences of nurses being mentored. These include avoiders – those who are neither physically nor emotionally accessible, and destroyers/ criticizers, mentors who in various ways undermine their mentee. To these I would add those whose motivation to take on the mentor role might be more related to enhancing their own power and advancing their own cause, those who show little respect for the differing views of others or, more simply, those who are unable to set aside their own agenda in order to pay attention to others.

The hope enshrined in making the introductory workshop a two-way process of selection is not dissimilar to any other organization using an induction phase. In providing the opportunity, you hope that those who display attitudes which make them unsuitable for the role will see this for themselves, and quietly withdraw, sparing the selectors any further trouble. For an example of what not to do when this doesn't happen, there is a long history in medicine of avoiding the de-selection of unsuitable doctors early in their career, opting instead to sign them up and move them on, so that they become someone else's problem, sparing the assessors the embarrassment of confrontation.

In the workshops, some participants of course displayed occasional toxic behaviours; after all, we are only human. In addition though, some members displayed behaviours which were much more overtly unhelpful to others – depression, agendas of obvious anger towards medicine and the world in general, and the sort of constant, overwhelming disapproval which is hard for any group to bear. In the event, only two of these applied to join the project, and this was quickly dealt by suggesting that, in the first instance, they received some mentoring for themselves.

But some other behaviours could not be so clearly categorized. There were participants who *appeared* as rigid, concrete thinkers, or arrogant and bombastic, or opinionated – but other participants in their group managed to work with them without any obvious sign of difficulty, so on what basis could it be said that they were unlikely to become effective mentors? Until the work had begun, no real assessment could be made, which brought, for the first time ever, some sympathy with the 'sign 'em up and move 'em on' method of de-selection.

Other themes emerged in reviewing the learning. The experience brought a clearer recognition that local *context* influences both perception of the mentoring task and its outcome. The role and function of mentors can be strongly determined by the organizational context, as the literature review shows, but in general practice it can be governed by local conditions, and the agenda which is uppermost in a participant's own mind. For example, some of the GP educators who attended the workshops were preoccupied with the need to construct and deliver relevant programmes of continuing education to their local population of doctors, and construed the mentor's role as one which would further this objective.

This might explain some of the confusion of terminology over the word 'mentor' abounding in general practice, and added a third level to the context of mentoring, so that a formulation phase needed to consider organizational, local, and individual contexts.

A further theme in the learning review was to do with *nurture*. The learning from the workshops showed clearly that the process of becoming a mentor involved being sufficiently nurtured oneself, further evidence for Winnicott's[22] view that one must receive nurture and support oneself to be able to offer it to others. The readiness with which the majority of the participants entered into the Reflective Cycle, and wanted more of the experience of shared reflection, emphasized the need to provide continuing developmental education for the mentor team as a source for their own nurturing.

A more personal reflection came from observing how, in the introductory workshops, my working relationship with intending mentors reflected that of their own with their mentee, a reflection which brought an unconscious realization into conscious knowledge, and made it available to be used. As the work progressed, my own role of 'mentor to the mentors' could be referred to, and explored as a model of a developing relationship. My point of contact was not with mentees, but with the mentors themselves, and their needs and interests were paramount. From her work supervising teams of caseworkers in the helping professions, Mattinson[23] concluded that relationships between workers and supervisors work best when they are not seen as discrete, but form a seamless web stretching into the extended network, an echo of Balint's[24] view of actively using the doctor–patient relationship to understand more about the process of the consultation. Rather than work at a distance from the mentor team, the 'supervisor' needed to create a good working relationship with the mentors, and strive towards establishing a trusting and supportive learning environment, so that they in turn could create something similar with their mentee.

The next telling phase would be the establishment phase, when we would discover how the early experience of the mentor team working with their mentees, and using the Reflective Cycle, would uphold the reasonable accuracy of the holistic model, reveal fault lines or, alternatively, show the need for a total redefinition of a mentoring intervention.

References

1 Freeman R. 1997 Towards effective mentoring in general practice. *British Journal of General Practice*, **47**, 457–60

2 Freeman R. 1994 Mentoring in general practice. *Journal of Education for General Practice*, **7**(2), 112–18

3 Quote taken from data gathered in the pre-pilot phase of the South Thames (West) Mentor Research Project, January 1995

4 Lomax P. 1995 Action research for professional practice. *British Journal of In-Service Education*, **21**(1), 49–51

5 Leff J. 1985 Unpublished seminar, Tavistock Clinic, London, July

6 Freeman R. 1997 An earlier summary appears in Chapter 6: Mentoring in general practice. In *Mentoring – The New Panacea?* (ed. Stephenson J.). Peter Francis Publishers

7 Kolb D. 1984 *Experiential Learning: Experience as a Source of Learning and Development.* Prentice Hall, Englewood Cliffs, New Jersey

8 Griffiths M. and Tann S. 1992 Using reflective practice to link personal and public theories. *Journal of Education for Teaching,* **18**(1), 69–84

9 Carruthers J. 1993 In *Return of the Mentor – Strategies for Workplace Learning* (eds Caldwell B. and Carter E.A.) Falmer Press, London

10 Levinson K., Darrow C., Klein E., Levinson M. and McKee B. 1978 *Seasons of a Man's Life.* Alfred A. Knopf, New York

11 Erikson E. 1950 *Childhood and Society.* Norton, New York

12 Morle K.M.F. 1990 Mentorship – a case of the Emperor's New Clothes – or a rose by any other name? *Nurse Education Today,* **10**, 66–9

13 Smail D. 1984 *Illusion and Reality – The Meaning of Anxiety.* J.M. Dent, London

14 Stephenson J (ed.) 1997 *Mentoring – the New Panacea?* Peter Francis Publishers

15 Balint M. 1964 *The Doctor, his Patient, and the Illness,* 2nd edn. Churchill Livingstone, London

16 Rogers C. 1980 *A Way of Being.* Houghton Mifflin, Boston

17 Burnard P. 1994 *Counselling Skills for Health Professionals,* 2nd edn. Chapman and Hall, London

18 Daloz L.A. 1987 *Effective Teaching and Mentoring.* Jossey-Bass, San Francisco, London

19 Egan G. 1994 *The Skilled Helper,* 5th edn. Brooks Cole, Pacific Grove CA

20 Op cit p.164

21 Darling, L.A. 1985 What to do about toxic mentors. *The Journal of Nursing Administration,* **15**(5), 43–4

22 Winnicott D. 1965 *Maturational Processes and the Facilitating Environment.* Hogarth Press, London

23 Mattinson J. 1975 *The Reflection Process in Casework Supervision.* Tavistock Institute of Human Relations, London

24 Balint M., ibid

4

Mentoring in practice

'The web of our life is a mingled yarn, good and ill together'
(*All's Well That Ends Well* Act 4 Scene 3)

Using the medium of the second training tier – the mentor support groups, and the plenary workshops – this chapter follows the progress made in the first year of the mentor's life as they took up their role, and discusses some of the themes that preoccupied mentors as their work developed. The data used here to illustrate themes and concepts come from three sources. The first was the reflective journal kept by the project leader to note learning themes and developing ideas in the groups and workshops. This journal was later analysed, and then compared with the second source, the content of semi-structured interviews with individual mentors in the first year of their mentor life. Occasionally group sessions were recorded, and material derived from their transcription is used as the third source.

Parallels are drawn between the important initial establishing phase of the mentor's relationship with their mentee, and that of myself as leader, similarly establishing a working relationship with the mentor teams as facilitator and leader of their support groups and plenary workshops. A consideration of the nature of this leadership role begins the descriptive account of the mentor's experience of using the Reflective Cycle, and putting holistic mentoring into practice.

Mentoring mentors – establishing a leadership role

Making bold statements about the need for ongoing development for mentors themselves begs the question of who takes on this developmental role with a mentor team. Some observers of our mentor scheme have commented that this aspect of developing the mentor team is the ideal, the 'gold standard' as one colleague put it, a role which can be dispensed with, particularly when mentors are likely to be self-sufficient practitioners and able to work constructively on their own, or available support resources are limited. However, our collective experience shows that as the project developed from its implementation phase, into a larger, ongoing regional scheme, the role of a designated leader with both the relevant knowledge and skills, and allocated time to pay full attention to mentoring activity, became a critical factor in maintaining the impetus of the project, and monitoring the effectiveness of its work.

Of course it is necessary to cut the coat according to the cloth, but the corporate experience shows that to invest resources in a helmsman (or woman) who can actively steer the project along its declared course, and develop its unforeseen potential, pays a good return. At the very least it ensures that mentees receive the best possible service from their peers, and it wins the confidence of the paymasters. Finding the right helms-person, a suitable mentor for the mentors as it were, is more problematic, and falls, it seems, between expediency, availability, and enthusiasm for the task – the latter being a definite bonus, but not perhaps a requirement. For readers poised to fall into either category, some aspects of my own experience are shared in this chapter. Another reason for including some comments on the experience is that, in the early stages of the mentor scheme's life, my own evolving role as the scheme leader mirrored the requirements of the mentor with their mentee. Like the mentors, my first tasks were to create an open and supportive environment in which to begin the work, to promote trust and confidence in our developing relationship, and to focus attention on a working agenda. I could present a confident and purposeful role model from my own resource and experience in order to achieve this, but my leadership would also need authority, and from where would that be derived?

Weber's[1] concept of authority distinguishes between three types – *traditional*, *legal-rational*, and *charismatic*. *Traditional* authority arises when a person is part of a group which has traditionally enjoyed authority. To some extent, my professional role within the postgraduate general practice deanery team might allow such a claim, but in this context it could not be assumed.

Charismatic authority Weber saw as arising from the individual's use of symbols of knowledge, a type of mystical knowledge, a somewhat different definition from the common notion of charisma as being associated with personal power and charm. Here it seemed I might be in with a chance; in working with mentors I consciously used my knowledge of developmental psychology, drawing on concepts which, for a discipline like medicine, placed a long way from the social sciences, might appear as arcane knowledge, particularly as my tendency to use myths as analogies is already obvious to readers.

Weber's third category of authority, *legal-rational*, is derived from the administrative framework of the organization. As such, in a bureaucratic structure, the authority to act autonomously, to give orders and enforce compliance, is seen as residing in the office, not the incumbent. Again, I could claim some authority from my formal adviser role within the organizational structure, but this would be of limited value given that taking on the role of a mentor was a voluntary activity, an optional role, not one taken up on the direction of the Postgraduate Dean of General Practice as head of an organization. Indeed, in some of the previous mentor schemes described in Chapter 3, mentees had been difficult to recruit precisely because they perceived the mentors as acting on their legal-rational authority, part of an authoritarian regional bureaucracy. Potential mentor project leaders would be wise to give thought to how their mentor team will perceive the nature of their authority.

Whilst Weber's three categories are useful in relation to organizations, they are confined by his perception of authority as being *external* – power bestowed by an organization, or by insider knowledge. This externally given power allows individuals to be *seen* as designated leaders. Many organizations and institutions convey the message of delegated power through external labelling – bigger and more sumptuous offices for the leaders, car-parking space which is marked out with the designated authority of the car's driver and reserved for their exclusive use, labels on office doors which declare the occupant to be a 'Head of . . .' or 'Director of . . .'; but few leaders can survive on these external labels alone. Initially, members of a team are prepared to accept the external authority and allow their leader an opportunity to perform, but simultaneously they are concerned to test the leader's ability to hold to their leadership role when faced with the challenges and confrontations arising from their interaction with members of their team.[2] For leadership to stand this test of application, a further dimension of authority is required, that of *internal* authority. This further dimension is less easily encapsulated in description, resting as it does in part on the leader's inner strength to withstand negative challenges to their leadership, and on their personal ability to inspire and motivate others. As my leadership role owed little to externally given authority, effective leadership of the mentor project was more likely to be grounded in my own personal, inner authority, the ability to act constructively on an inner belief.

It has always seemed to me that general practitioners are uncomfortable with the notion of authority, although they have so much of it in their working role, and even less comfortable with the concept of power, so that, for example, in continuing education, more neutral-sounding titles like 'facilitator' are preferred to ones which imply authority. Perhaps, like people the world over, the thought of powerful leadership is linked to the shadow side of power, and recalls experiences of being led by those driven by the pursuit of personal power, determined to maintain total control over members of their working team, operating highly authoritarian structures which either serve to stifle the creative energy of their team, or ensure that anything good which comes from their team is directly attributed to them, and used to advance their own power. Being the victim of negative power is a crippling experience, and makes more elusive the conscious thought of power as a positive force, directed not at the advancement of self, but the advancement of others.

In their comprehensive study of what distinguished effective from ineffective leaders, Bennis and Nanus,[3] seeking to elicit the personal dimensions of leadership, stated categorically that:

'. . . leadership is modelled on . . . power'

but went on to define the nature of that power as being the

'basic energy needed to initiate and sustain action, or, to put it another way, the capacity to translate intention into reality and sustain it'

and stressed the positive aspect of using such power appropriately:

'Leadership is the wise use of this power: transformative *leadership'* (p. 17).

As this mentor project moved through the stage of intent into sustaining reality, and at times struggled to sustain intention in the face of competing demands, this concept of transformative leadership became increasingly meaningful. And acutely relevant to the implementation phase was the Bennis and Nanus's further prediction that, to succeed in this transformative power, leaders need vision:

'vision is the commodity of leaders and power their currency'(p. 18).

The introductory workshops had offered a vision of mentoring. Those doctors who became mentors had shared sufficiently in the vision to give their initial commitment towards it becoming a reality. For this reality to be fulfilled, the support groups required a style of leadership that would maintain the mentor's energy and commitment to follow a process of enquiry and experimentation, towards making a shared vision reality. In this important establishing phase, it was clearly essential that I, as leader, kept the vision in view. In the early stages, before the scheme became more firmly established, this meant containing my own uncertainties until such time as we had sufficient data to make a first evaluation and discover whether the vision was at least partly realizable.

Goffman[4] sums up this leadership predicament nicely:

'Similarly, if the individual offers to the others a product, or service, they will often find that during the interaction there is no time and place immediately available for eating the pudding that the proof can be found in' (p. 14).

For more about proving the pudding, see Chapters 6 and 7. In the meantime, my leadership authority rested not on any hierarchical strength, but on transformative power – the power to help transform the experience of the mentors working with their mentees. In the mentor support groups, the stages of the learning cycle – reflection on concrete experience, conceptualization, and further implementation – needed to be worked around, so that the mentors' new learning was consolidated, and became a source of accessible and usable knowledge.

Starting work – opening Pandora's box

To share with readers of this book the early experience of the mentors as they began their work replicates to some extent concerns about confidentiality in the mentoring relationship. In the support groups, the mentor's reflection on their experience rightly took into account the ethics surrounding confidential information. Initially, this was a difficult dilemma for the mentors, as they juggled their own need to share and discuss issues with each other and their professional responsibility to preserve the confidentiality of their session with the mentee. It had been made clear from the introductory workshops that the function of the mentor support groups was to focus on the *mentor's* experience, by reflecting on their own action and responses to their mentee's agenda – the 'concrete experience'. From this the support group had a shared learning base from which to conceptualize, and develop strategies for further interventions. After some initial uncertainties, and testing out, the mentor team learned to relate the general themes of the content of their session – to place their own actions in context – without divulging the content in detail, or revealing any identifying features of their mentee. In essence, the mentee's story was infinitely less interesting to us than the mentor's story, for it was they who had the focus of attention, in order to learn.

In this chapter, the same maxim is upheld – it is the themes which emerged as the context of the mentor's experience which are commented upon; where data from the group sessions are used to illustrate these themes, permission to share these with readers has been given by the protagonists involved.

All of the themes discussed here have a unifying concept, which appears as the nature of anxiety. In the establishing phase of the work, anxiety was uppermost, naturally so given that mentors were starting a new task, and also had to carry the uncertainty of their mentee about the whole process. But as the work moved into its ongoing phase, the anxiety grew less intense, and then the primary focus shifted onto how the mentor's own personal and professional identity might be influenced by the role, and by their work with each other in the support groups. Anxiety never quite went away, but the nature of it changed, it grew more manageable, and settled at an appropriate level, for as one experienced mentor said, after over 2 years of mentoring:

'I don't ever *not* feel anxious – after all each time you meet with a mentee you are fired up – but there's a difference now. The anxiety gives me a buzz; it's a positive source of energy, it's exciting'.

That, of course was much further on in the story, so how was the anxiety expressed in those first few weeks of face-to-face work?

Safety in structure

Early in the life of the support groups, both the mentor teams were pre-occupied with the structures surrounding their mentoring work, represented by the scheme's administrative frameworks.

Had I opted to aspire to being a charismatic leader, I would have responded more fittingly to this preoccupation, with sensitivity and patient concern, calmly reiterating the use of various administrative forms; instead, I struggled to repress my own mounting impatience and irritation. I had spent much time and thought to provide straightforward and clear structures for mentoring, and had devised the Reflective Cycle as a further means of structuring the initial process of mentoring sessions. Yet here we were going backwards (it seemed), spending precious time not on what they actually *did* with their mentee, but on questions such as: who took the initiative in making contact with the mentee?; should you wait for the mentee to make contact, as a test of their motivation, or should mentors actively make the first move? And it was clear, as all eyes turned towards me, that they were awaiting direction from me on this point – again seeking structure.

Under such scrutiny I too began to feel anxious, I caught myself skimming through my own notes to confirm the accuracy of my answers to their questions, and inside I felt that I had failed them after all. The clarity of the administrative framework, the apparent enthusiasm of the introductory workshops was all a fantasy, another case of the *Emperor's New Clothes*. Then, gradually, through the mist of my own anxiety, I began to see that the mentor's need to check and re-check the observable, safe administrative framework was a vehicle by which they could alleviate some of their anxiety about beginning the mentoring task. It echoed the experience of those mentors in other projects who, faced with personal issues, took flight into educational planning, using an educational contract as an overt, safe, structure.

In her seminal text describing how organizations defend themselves against feeling anxious, Menzies-Lyth[5] discusses how certain features of the nursing service in a large hospital could be viewed as institutional structures which functioned to defend nursing staff against anxiety. When student nurses first came onto the wards, and began nursing for real, experiencing the full weight of patients' anxieties, and carrying responsibility for their care, they experienced overwhelming anxiety. The hospital avoided this anxiety by constantly moving nurses around, only allowing nurses short, restricted spells on one ward before moving them on, thus preventing them becoming too intimate with patients.

It was natural for mentors, faced with a new and unknown task, to feel anxious; indeed it was appropriate that they should feel so, and it indicated their serious commitment to their mentee. Part of this anxiety, which became more evident later, was the very continuing intimacy of an ongoing mentoring relationship. Unlike the 10-minute consultation, which avoids the exposure of time, the mentors had to manage the structure of their session for at least an hour.

Like nurses, mentors sought ways to alleviate their anxiety in the structures of the project, thereby dispelling it by following ritual instructions. All mentors came to these groups with their *Handbook* – in itself astoundingly unusual. Doctors generally dispense with written protocols, and frequently arrive for educational events without relevant course documentation which they have 'forgotten', 'mislaid', swear they have never received, but most probably have thrown in the waste paper bin unread. Perhaps carrying the 'book' gave additional confidence, in much the same way that Bion[6] describes work groups who needed a symbolic bible – sometimes the group leader – in which, (or from whom) 'answers' could be sought which would stave off feelings of uncertainty and anxiety.

During some previous work in group dynamics, when I had probably felt just as much at sea, and confused about what was going on, I had built on concepts of group development[7] to formulate my own understanding of the stages of group life,[8] similar to stages of personality development – infancy, adolescence and adulthood. In 'infancy' when the group is newly formed, and still establishing its identity, members will look upon the leader much as a parent, and seek from them fairly constant feeding via constant stating and re-stating of the task, the structure of the task, and its relationship to the outside world. Only later, as the group establishes a collective identity, do they recapture their adult confidence in their ability to understand the task, and how to set about it. At this time in the mentor team's life they looked towards me for direction and instruction, the 'parent' figure providing some structure and certainty in the unknown task.

But, when on the job, and working with the mentee, did the mentor's natural anxiety show through, and hinder their establishing a rapport with their mentee and hearing their agendas?

Containing anxiety

This is perhaps a good point to recall the story of *Pandora's Box* (or, at least, the beginning of it, because the end of the story comes in Chapter 6):

Pandora was created by Hephaestus from the moulded figure of a perfect young girl, to which he gave the power of speech. Receiving from Athene the spirit of life, and from Aphrodite beguiling beauty, her future was promising. However, Hermes intervened and instilled deceit, wantonness and foolishness into her breast. Forgetting dire warnings never to accept gifts from Zeus, Epimetheus, overwhelmed by her beauty, took Pandora (meaning 'all gifts') as his wife.

Lovely, but empty headed, Pandora appears as decorous but useless. Left alone one day, bored and disconsolate in her husband's absence, she came upon the fascinating jar her husband had so firmly forbade her to touch. When cautiously lifting the lid to peer curiously inside, a cloud of stinging, biting creatures flew out, covering Pandora and Epimetheus who had come rushing over in answer to Pandora's terrified cry. The creatures vanished. She had let out every ill, trouble and sin known to the world.[9,10]

Furthermore, it seemed that foolish Pandora had allowed all her creatures to fly direct into the orbit of general practice mentors, who came to their support groups and regaled us with their experiences of early meetings in which they were deluged by the number of problems their mentees presented to them:

'it was like sitting under an avalanche – I staggered home and had two large Scotches and started to write up my notes – and then I thought – where the hell do we begin?'

'Everywhere in her life she has problems – and she gave me the lot, all of them, inside 2 hours'

However, when mentors outlined the *nature* of the problems, no evidence was given of the sick doctors they had so feared in the introductory workshops, who would unleash upon them the evils of the medical world – no mentees came with awful entrenched problems of drug addiction, unethical behaviours with patients, suicidal states, madness, or the like. In fact, the ills and troubles which flew around the mentors were pretty familiar stuff – problems with partners in the practice, the distress of a pending complaint, the misery of failing the MRCGP. To further confound us, from the notes of my reflective journal which recorded the content of these early support groups, comes an example of a mentor who, despite being told not to open the jar, could not resist the thought of doing so:

B (the mentor) drops the bombshell into the group that his mentee had asked for help with his unhappy marriage – could the mentor meet his wife and explain to her how demanding the work of a general practitioner was? I am conscious of some anxious looks in my direction and could read the thoughts that gathered like clouds over their heads – what will she think about this? Did she not say in the training workshops that married agendas should be kept out of it? What will she say/do now?

   B, however, is totally unconcerned. He wonders if it would not be more productive to see husband and wife together. There is an audible gasp. 'No, no', the group cry in unison, surely this isn't mentoring. B asks, 'why not?' – it is a partnership, like any other partnership. Underneath this mentor's quiet exterior is a watchful, insightful inner eye, I know it. And, sure enough, he poses the question to his peers – just suppose these two were in practice together? And, if they were, and they both asked to be mentored, what would other mentors do?

Surely it would be absolutely normal to mentor them. 'Yes', said the group, but not at the same time, nor together, because our job is to help him tell his wife that her demands are unreasonable (interestingly, they all assume that the wife is unreasonable . . .). I ask, 'what does this mentee want out of his mentoring?'

The group discuss this, and conclude that he wants his mentor as an ally – not against his wife, as they first thought, but against the overwhelming demand of the job, someone to help him claim some space for himself.

And so it seemed that mentors were less concerned with the potential *nature* of the mentee's problems, than with making them *manageable* through organizing their disclosure. Other examples from mentors told a similar story, when they talked of being deluged by problems, they were not, as I had first thought, fearing the content, but rather being rendered useless by the sheer volume of issues. The root of their anxiety lay not in opening the jar and releasing evils, but in being unable to marshal them into some sort of manageable agenda so that they might be addressed.

On more than one occasion, I suggested that it was not the *mentor's* job to put problems into some sort of order, it was the *mentee's*. In saying to the mentee:

'there are a lot of issues and problems which you have identified in this session – where do you want us to start? Would you like to prioritize them, so that we can work our way through your agenda?',

the responsibility for the agenda was once again firmly with the mentee, who in turn took responsibility for deciding which of many issues they themselves wanted to address first.

It sounded simple, yet this sort of utterance was always received with relief by the mentor teams. It was clear that they themselves had not immediately seen where the responsibility for the ordering of a deluge lay, and gradually I saw a link between this and their professional role as doctors. We were still in the world of myth, but the myth had to do with 'cure' rather than 'containment'. In their medical role, problems were there to be cured, or, second best, managed in ways which alleviated their impact on the patient's life. The concept of 'containing' problems through acknowledging their presence, and clarifying their impact on an individual's life, guiding the person with the problem to find their own way to resolve or ameliorate them, was naturally alien. The mentors totally accepted this in their head, as they had in the introductory workshops, but in their heart they were healers, and almost instinctively leaned towards finding a cure, a solution for 'dis-ease'.

The experience of being deluged revealed another aspect of managing the mentor's role, one which had to do with accepting that it was not possible to change the unchangeable. For a few of the mentees, their life pattern was one of constant anxiety; they had, as it were, been born with problems. This introduced the need to differentiate between those transient episodes of anxiety which occur in response to various life events, and those for whom anxiety was a way of life, like a chronic pain. For these colleagues, the mentor's task became one of helping them to manage their anxiety better, an aspect captured by Smail[11] when writing about the language of anxiety:

'That is not to say one can do nothing about the reasons for the [other person's] dread, only that the solution to the "problems" they pose is not to be found in somehow juggling the individual's interpretation or perception of his or her experience. Though such juggling may be useful and validly form part of a process in which people begin to gain a subjective purchase on their predicament, it is, in the end, their actual embodied relations with their circumstances which count. Even then new experience does not obliterate old . . . thus people whose insecurity is fundamental to their experience almost certainly will never become fundamentally secure, though they may come to be able to acknowledge their insecurity in ways which mitigate its intensity and minimize the effects it has on the actual conduct of their lives' (p. 90).

The task of the mentor lay in offering other perspectives on the mentee's 'problem', and exploring its relationship to the rest of life – containment not cure. For more than a few mentors, experiencing this distinction was an illuminating learning experience:

'I realized very quickly, in our second meeting it was, I am not here to solve. I am here to listen. I hold up a mirror and wipe the mist off – that's it – a de-misted mirror!'

And what was the mentor's experience of using the Reflective Cycle – a strategy which was, after all, designed to reduce the mentor's early anxiety, and boost their initial confidence?

Using (or not) the Reflective Cycle

As has been said before, all of the mentors shared various feelings of vulnerability when first meeting their mentee. Anxious to appear confident and purposeful, they were acutely aware of the critical nature of their first two meetings. Some mentors had felt themselves to be very much 'on trial', and, while others had felt an immediate positive bond between themselves and their mentee, everyone had experienced it as a testing time. Although it was this anticipated factor which gave rise to the design of the Reflective Cycle as a supportive strategy, nevertheless it was useful at this stage to remind mentors that their feelings of vulnerability were shared by 'professional' mentors working in disciplines where professional one-to-one interventions were the main task of the organization, and accepted patterns of 'in house' supervision exist.[12]

To counter these feelings, most of the mentors had used the developmental cycle, although some who were confident of their interviewing skills decided not to use it:

'after the introductory workshop, I thought, well . . . I've spent a lifetime interviewing people . . . I've got my own ideas of how to approach this . . .'

but, for some, this confidence waned as the mentoring session began:

'in fact, after the introductions it was a bit like that book – you know – what do you say when you have said "hello"? After a bit of wandering around, I thought, "oh well, we'll give it a try", and I got the cycle out and showed it to M (the mentee) and he seemed quite interested in working around it'.

Another who had not intended to use it gave a delightful, humorous account of how his uncertainty got the better of him:

'I set off for the session, looking forward to it, quite excited actually . . . I got there early, in good time, so sat in the car park for a bit – and as the time got closer all the confidence I set off with ebbed away and formed in puddles around my feet. I was determined not to use any cycle, after all we are doctors, been at this interviewing thing for years – and then I sat there and thought . . . well, perhaps I might . . . then I got in a panic because I thought, did I even bring the *Handbook* with me?, so that after all I was nearly late as I ransacked the car, found the *Handbook* and rifled desperately through the pages to get the Cycle into my head'.

For those who did use the Reflective Cycle, their motivation to do so came in part it seemed from the responsibility of working with their peers, and their overwhelming concern that they should offer them quality time. Using the Cycle meant that the usefulness of the session was not left to chance:

'using it showed the mentee that I took this seriously, that I had aims for our sessions'

and this lowered the mentor's own anxieties:

'it is not that I am not anxious (as a mentor) – of course I am – but I was more worried about what would happen if there seemed nothing to talk about – if we both sat there staring at each other, each waiting for the other to kick off'.

Other mentors used the Cycle in their second mentoring interview, finding that the first one was very much a getting-to-know session, with information about professional backgrounds and interests being exchanged as a prelude to work:

'in the first interview you are testing each other out – perhaps they need to find out if they can trust you'

but all those who did use it agreed that it served them well as a route map from which to begin their journey of exploration, a map which could be discarded once their relationship gained its own sense of direction:

'at first they are unsure – they sort of sit there waiting to be told what to do – like all doctors, that's what they're used to. But by the second session they come with their lists, and their agendas, ready to get started'.

Towards the end of this establishing phase mentors became less pre-occupied with managing the content and structure of mentoring sessions, and more concerned with how they used themselves in the relationship. There was much discussion about 'getting it right' for the mentee, and getting it right centred on increasing their knowledge of the mentoring process, and developing skills that would offer their mentee something more than a supportive conversation. It brought to the fore skills employed in fully attending to the mentee's agenda, showing verbally and non-verbally a non-judgmental interest and concern in the mentee's professional life. Mentors developed the art of asking open-ended questions to explore events, and they took a fresh look at the skill of listening – a skill which previously they thought they had possessed in full measure as they used it daily in the consultation; but, by examining their experience of active listening as they responded to the mentee's agenda, the mentors began to sense a different quality of listening, and through this came to see that quality listening in itself offered a means of containing issues brought by their mentee. In their mentoring sessions, they learned to listen at two levels, for what was not said, as well as the words that came, and this required their utmost attention.

The mentor teams then began to listen to each other in the support workshops at this different level and, on the whole, moved away from doctor-mode in which one listened in order to prescribe, and developed the art of listening and reflecting upon what they had heard, before speaking themselves. Many mentors were struck by this different quality of listening:

'I am amazed at what happens if you simply listen – really listen, just sit, and be.'

In the endeavour to 'get it right' another important theme emerged, and that had to do with boundaries. Mentors were concerned to convey to their mentee that they were not experts, but at the same time they did have sufficient experience and knowledge to contain the agenda and help the mentee move on, forward from where they currently were in their professional life. The mentors wanted to engender a sense of empathy, to 'join' the mentee, stand alongside them, and in doing so they tested out the boundary between using their own experience to convey identification, but not taking over the mentee's agenda with tales of their own:

'I thought it would be good to tell him [the mentee] how I felt when in this situation (a patient complaint) and what I did to cope with it . . . but after I finished there was dead silence. I realize, looking back, I probably went too far – what I mean is, there's a difference between saying how the same situation made you feel, and telling someone how you handled it, and implying that they should do the same'

. . . a nice example of what Rogers[13] implies by empathic listening.

Another aspect of managing boundaries was the mentor's developing confidence in moving between the three components of holistic mentoring – continuing education, personal development and professional development. Once the concept of containing problems, not curing them, had been grasped it helped mentors feel more confident in using open questions to explore life events with their mentee, and this in turn encouraged mentees to bring a wide range of issues to their working agendas, such as are summarized here:

Continuing education included structural issues such as identifying educational aims, and how these could be realized, together with planning a programme of continuing education over the forthcoming year, and more immediate issues like passing the MRCGP exam.

Personal issues included developing coping strategies for work-related stress, within which the immediate presentation of personal stress, or managing the boundary between work and home life, and the stress of being in conflict with partners, was explored.

Professional development included strategic planning for a future work life, setting some life goals and drawing up action plans to realize them, together with infinitely more immediate issues of partnership problems, personal disillusionment with the role of general practice, and practice management and organization.

This range of issues brought by the mentees portrays the importance of having mentors with a range of skills which enable them to respond flexibly, and move between the three components. Some of the skills employed are described here under each of the three components, beginning with *continuing education*. The mentors had previously thought this area of education to be familiar and fairly easy, but their developing experience showed clearly that each mentoring relationship was very individual, and potentially complex, even when it was the vehicle for the exploration of an 'ordinary' topic such as continuing education.

A very few mentees came to their mentor with clear educational agendas, for which, it seemed, they wanted their mentor's confirmation that they were 'right'. They were resistant to the mentor's attempts to facilitate further learning, preferring to remain within their own existing paradigms of thought and action. More came with a less fixed educational agenda, and sought more from their mentor in the way of exploring possible alternatives, clearly using the mentoring opportunity to review beliefs and knowledge uncritically assimilated and carried forward from earlier educational experiences. This frequently had the 'knock-on' effect of challenging the mentor to review their own assimilated beliefs (but in the protected space of the support group). Working within the frameworks of adult learning, mentors explored the use of educational agreements, and personal learning plans[14] in their mentoring sessions, finding that mentees who came with educational issues high on the agenda benefited most from the mentor's impartiality in discussing how learning needs had been identified. In addition to working out 'wants and needs' with the mentee, the mentor's neutrality made it possible to suggest that, at times, the mentee was over-learning, choosing knowledge areas with which they were reasonably familiar to confirm present knowledge, as opposed to taking risks with areas of unfamiliar learning and perhaps in areas which were resisted – for example, learning to use a computer. The use of explorative, non-judgmental questioning, by a neutral peer who had no personal investment in the learning outcomes of their mentee, made it more possible to move towards a view of learning as continuous improvement, rather than a 'one-off' occasional event to fill a gap in knowledge. Addressing continuing education as an ongoing professional activity[15] extended the mentee's thinking to beyond the next upcoming seminar, or five-day course, to see its position in the wider scheme of their professional development.

These educational agendas demanded from the mentor skills in assisting their mentees to articulate their educational wants and needs, to help them formulate a learning plan, then support the plan as it unfolded, monitoring its progress, and defining outcomes. Described generally as facilitation, it was not always easy, for a number of reasons, one of which is eloquently identified by Egan:[16]

'How long does helping take? . . . the helper should move as quickly through the stages and steps needed by the client . . . Beginning helpers often dally too long in stage one, not merely because they have a deep respect for the necessity of relationship development and problem clarification, but because they either do not know how to move on, or fear doing so. [Some] clients may be able to move quickly to action, their helper . . . should be able to move with them' (p. 45).

The mentor teams were at the beginning of their own learning curve, and were aware that they too had to address gaps in knowledge or understanding. Working with the educational component pushed mentors to read around issues of self-directed learning, and then to discuss their understanding with peers in their support group, whilst making explicit requests to me to address aspects of educational facilitation in the developmental workshops, when all the teams came together to address their own identified learning agendas.

However, as Brookfield[17] points out it is all too easy to see the job of a facilitator as one concerned solely with assisting adults to meet those educational needs which they themselves perceive and express as meaningful and important. Facilitator is usually taken to mean someone who assists, rather than directs adults along learning pathways towards achieving a more fulfilled state of being. Unfortunately, the word is too often used inaccurately to describe someone whose sole task is to initiate discussion, or locate possible individuals, or material resources to aid the learner, and then bows out, taking no responsibility for what happens afterwards, and certainly not for the realization of learning outcomes.

This is a flawed, if comfortable perception of an uncomfortable task, for a true facilitator points out the contradictions in a learning plan, or a statement made, is capable of suggesting more complex alternatives, and can prompt critical reflection on an action. Facilitators enter into painful, uncomfortable scrutinies of assumptions on which statements and actions are based, they question the values which underpin behaviour, and generally make a nuisance of themselves. The skills defined as necessary for this unpopular role are equally difficult to achieve, being those of constructive confrontation, and appropriate, well timed challenges to the status quo. They are skills constantly required by holistic mentors, albeit at different levels, ranging from confronting abstract concepts to confronting an individual in a personal interaction.

An example of the former is the experience of mentors who, in the process of exploring an educational issue, confronted the false divide between thinking and feeling, a divide begun in medical school when the student is inducted into the ethos of medicine, and part of the hidden curriculum of medical school commented on by Marinker[18] with searing insight:

'there runs throughout the process of medical education an assumption that thinking and feeling are not only separate human functions, but actually that each is inimical to the other' (p. 452).

The confrontation was made possible by the mentors moving around the Reflective Cycle exploring with mentees their educational experience. Here mentors found that at times they needed to deviate from the educational pathway and make a diversion into personal support. This served as a test of applied theory, when the flexibility of holistic mentoring, with the mentor moving backwards and forwards between components, was tried out.

The legacy of negative learning experienced in medical education for some mentees surfaced when exploring with their mentor the nature of their blocks to learning, which in turn gave expression to the feelings which accompanied the event. These unexpressed feelings undermined rational thinking about present learning opportunities, one consequence of which, for example, is to defend against putting yourself back into a situation of shared learning, out of fear that once again your gaps in knowledge will be cruelly highlighted. Faced with such situations, mentors had to move to the dimension of personal support, to use their communication skills of listening, and sensitively exploring the feelings that accompanied uncomfortable learning events, before moving back again into the thinking component of the educational facilitator, drawing up an educational plan which might support the mentee to go out and give small group learning another try. In this they had a fair measure of success, because the fact of the mentor's continuing support and sole interest in their mentee created a supportive climate for their learning process.

When working in the area of *professional development*, mentors inevitably encouraged instances where their mentees' feelings about their professional life – both positive and negative – spilled over into their personal life and vice versa. The support groups were regularly used to check that boundaries were kept and that mentors were not inappropriately sliding, or being seduced by their mentee, into becoming surrogate trainer, academic tutor, or personal therapist, although occasional incursions were recognized, however, as part of the art of mentoring. Mentors discovered for themselves that making brief excursions across boundaries to work with feelings often enabled their mentee to think more clearly, and this in itself encouraged them to move more freely between the components of holistic mentoring, recognizing that such flexibility brought rewards.

For example, when mentors talked with doctors about their choice of career – both those at the start of their professional life as well as established practitioners facing another 15 years in practice – and explored what these doctors felt now about general practice, a range of feelings, including disillusionment and apathy about future professional life were brought out. Here, mentors found themselves using one of the six interventions described by Heron[19] as cathartic, to enable their mentee to discharge their anger, frustration, and occasionally their grief about the current state of their profession. Catharsis brings a sense of release; having discharged feelings, thinking re-asserts itself, but more successfully. The agenda of a future professional life could be addressed with more insight, and calm, and the positive aspects of practice rediscovered. For some mentors, working with their mentee in this way gave rise to their own needs; although they were diligent about not encroaching on their mentee's space, they themselves identified with many of the feelings expressed, and on occasions used the support groups for their own catharsis.

Nor could mentors leave out of this discussion the effect that professional life had on personal life. Asking about future hopes – where the doctor wanted to be in 5 years' time, elicited life goals that included a spouse, and children, or the intention to establish a family life. At times the conflicting hopes and desires of the mentee and their life partner came on to the agenda, and not uncommonly exposed feelings of resentment against the encroachment of professional life into personal life. Here again mentors moved between personal and professional issues, and here again it was to continue the debate on boundaries. How far should the mentor go? Should they actively explore, say, the mentee's fear that unless s/he could claim back some personal space from the overwhelming demand of clinical practice s/he will in 5 years' time be without a life partner? It was perhaps more in this area of holistic mentoring that mentors learned to handle the boundary between *investigating* a problem, and empathically *listening* to better understand it. Unlike secondary care, general practice works on the boundary of art and science, between conjecture and investigation. In practice, mentors began to sense the similar boundary that exists in mentoring, began to develop their intuitive feel for when to investigate an issue further and when, together with their mentee, speculate, drawing out 'what if' scenarios of the future.

More pragmatic skills were used too. Mentees who were young principals frequently asked their mentors for feedback on how they were doing. Feedback is a prerequisite of professional development, yet, having left their trainer behind, doctors establishing themselves in the profession found it difficult to locate peers who would listen to their handling of a patient, or staff problem, and offer some constructive feedback on how it was handled. For those mentors who were also trainers, the art of constructive feedback on performance was familiar, and it was they who helped their peer mentors in the support group to develop a planned approach to giving feedback. The independent status of the mentor also meant that they were asked for their opinion on practice management problems: delegating work, negotiating with health authorities, handling disciplinary and other staff problems. This introduced another layer of skills, of problem-solving techniques that lay within the framework of force-field analysis, where the future state is identified before looking at the current reality, and identifying the helping and hindering forces which prevent the future state being achieved. Mentors drew up action plans with their mentees to remove these hindrances, or to plan strategically to reduce them, and then work towards the desired outcome of improving practice management.

But, for the mentor team in whose geographical area 65% of doctors were single-handed practitioners, and predominantly of Asian origin, working on their mentees' professional development introduced another, paradoxical aspect of keeping boundaries. In addition to 'how far should one go?' came 'how much should one do?'. This extract from my field notes is an illustration:

All the group tell me they are deluged with practice problems – their mentees want additional hours for a nurse, extensions to their premises, more money from the health authority, and, to cap it all, one of them wants his mentor to arrange for him 3 months' sabbatical. In short, all the mentees want their mentor to fix it for them. And the group discussion mirrors precisely this – there is a lot of prescribing of solutions, and telling each other what they 'ought' and 'should' say to their mentees, and where the right answer to the questions can be found. After a while, M says 'wait a minute – we are all behaving like doctors'. She goes on to draw parallels between prescribing cures for patients and prescribing answers for mentees. What a prize this is – I had clumsily attempted something similar earlier, and been completely dismissed, and now M comes back to it, puts it beautifully, times it superbly, and gets their attention.

The group stops talking for a while, and appears to think about this, and then R thoughtfully tells us about spending time in the library finding out information for his mentee, and then he says: 'what I want to know is this – should it be 90% me and 10% him – or what should it be?'

Exactly – the question precisely. It did not take this team long to rediscover that they had been seduced into acting *for* their mentees, rather acting as a resource which would enable them to act for themselves. They discussed how to restore a healthier balance, one which came to rest at least on a 50–50 share base. But in an Eastern culture, gurus and mentors are fixers; they bear a closer resemblance to the mentors in American business who 'open doors' for their protégés, and use their influence and power to 'fix' the future for them. The expectation of the Asian mentees was of this nature, mentors with their greater power and influence would approach the health authority, and act as advocate, putting their case for their practice extension, or extra nurse, and pleading on their behalf. In developing the requisite mentor skills which facilitate others to act for themselves, these mentors realized that they had also to educate their mentees in the different nature of the mentoring relationship. And some mentees would never accept this empowering role – if the mentor could not fix it, they were redundant in their eyes, they could see no further use for their skills.

Comparing this experience with that of the mentor team working in very different circumstances south of the Thames shows a difference not as great as might be imagined. The mentor team in the South also struggled with how much of the action to take on, but their mentees seemed generally more receptive to the idea of shared responsibility.* Questions about action were answered more readily, for example, by using the mentoring session to role-play a forthcoming interview, particularly when it involved negotiation, or confrontation, providing a rehearsal and feedback session to the mentee on how to present themselves.

Finally, we came to the area of *personal support*, in which the mentors' fears of opening *Pandora's Box* were based, and firmly illustrated by this comment:

'mentoring isn't for sick doctors – I don't like all this psychological medicine stuff – we aren't therapists and that's not what the mentees want'.

In the event, once the mentors began work, the anxieties expressed about 'personal therapy' diminished rapidly and it was as if, having taken the lid off the jar, the evils that flew out were infinitely smaller than imagined. Mentors could indeed now see for themselves that personal therapy was not what their *mentees* wanted. In the first 2 years of the scheme, when 58 mentees came into it, only two were identified by mentors as having personal problems which would benefit from other, specifically personal

---

* Possible reasons for this difference are discussed in Chapter 8.

help. On these occasions, the mentors suggested other sources of help, and worked to ensure that the referral was made promptly, and sensitively. Most importantly, this did not bring to an end the mentoring relationship; it simply removed some aspects from the agenda.

Mentees wanted support, not psychology, as the summary of discussion themes show. They wanted support to manage the stress of the workplace, a chance to work out with their mentor some coping strategies, and to find ways of managing the boundaries between personal life and work life more effectively. Again mentors did some homework, and sharpened up on their knowledge of time management, and strategies for reducing stress. Not infrequently the mentor located some suitable workbook on these issues, and reviewed it with their mentee, discussing as they went the application of the ideas to general practice – shared learning. Within the mentor team were practitioners who themselves had made a particular study of stress management, and they were used as another, valuable resource in the mentor groups from which to develop skills and knowledge.

By far the most acute presentation in this personal area were the mentees' unhappy relationships with their partners in practice. As an earlier chapter commented, dysfunctional practices and difficult partners were a major source of stress. It was here that the mentor's ability to offer quality listening, without making value judgements, and to reflect back to their mentee what they had heard him or her say, proved its value. Checking the accuracy of their listening – 'this is what I have heard – is this what you said?' and acknowledging the distortion that can occur in translation, prompted, it seemed, further insight into considering how the actions and responses of the mentee might be viewed by their partners. Asking the open question, 'how do you think your partners view you?', moved the mentor skills into another of Heron's[20] categories, that of the catalytic intervention, in which the helper firmly, but empathically, prompts self-discovery.

Overall, the mentor teams were able to lay down their preoccupation with the dangers of personal therapy, finding themselves comfortable with the level of personal support offered to their mentees, and to each other in the support groups. But they were interested to discuss the nature of their previous anxiety, and one mentor put the locus for this very clearly, and in so doing resolved the problem left hanging in the air in the introductory workshops (referred to in Chapter 3):

'we think we know about psychotherapy or counselling – but we only see our patients for a few minutes. It's easy to think you can do it for – at the most – half an hour at the end of the surgery. We see our mentees time after time – a continuous relationship – it's a more intimate relationship and that's what our anxieties have been about'

In the reality of practice, the mentors found that they were not sought by those overwhelmed with personal difficulties, or those who had already made maladaptations to stress and resorted to alcohol or drugs. Mentoring implies purposeful professional development, and as such is unlikely to appeal to those who have already lost sight of their energy and ability to change. But whilst the holistic, developmental nature of the model is seen as essential to a framework of continuing professional development, mentors should be clear not only about those issues that fall outside their task, but know where to link in to other sources of knowledge and expertise. To this end, the scheme is slowly building a resource bank of individuals and organizations offering a variety of interventions – from stress counselling and aromatherapy to educational programmes, practice development, and routes to academic study – in order to respond creatively to the agenda of their mentees.

Reviewing the implementation phase of the mentor scheme, it appeared that the basic energy needed to initiate action, and the careful attention paid to developing a comprehensive support structure had paid off. There was a general feeling that the scheme was firmly grounded. The regular support groups, to which mentors willingly came, led to a harnessing of collective mentor experience, giving a consolidated, coherent view of the mentor's role in general practice, and providing the learning themes for the developmental workshops.

It appeared that the developmental cycle served its intended purpose, and, in its implementation, mentors sharpened known skills in listening, exploring, and reflecting on the content of their professional discussions with mentees. As the volume of work developed, other skills and knowledge areas were drawn in, so that, overall, mentors did move in step with their mentees as had been envisaged. Working in this paced way, the teams discovered the reality of acting as a mentor – that they did not need enormous stock piles of answers, and infinite wisdom, but instead the capacity of reflective judgement which works outside the boundaries of certain knowledge, giving up the need to 'know' in favour of exploring the reason why.

Like all good stories then, it may seem that all is set to end well. Heroes and heroines have overcome anxiety and difficulties, and have learnt a lot on the way towards their ultimate goal; the wind seems set for fair for the rest of the developmental voyage. As any realist knows, of course, all that really means is that there is trouble around the corner, and so it proved.

References

1 Weber M. 1947 *The Theory of Social and Economic Organization*. Free Press, New York
2 Freeman R. 1986 Leading from the edge management in general practice. *Horizons*, Issue 1, 39–42
3 Bennis W. and Nanus B. 1985 *Leaders – the Strategies for Taking Charge*. Harper and Row, New York
4 Goffman, E. 1959 *The Presentation of Self in Everyday Life*. Pelican, UK
5 Menzies-Lyth I. 1988 *Containing Anxiety in Institutions – Selected Essays*. Free Association Books, London
6 Bion W.R. 1961 *Experiences in Groups and Other Papers*. Tavistock, Basic Books, London
7 See for example Whitaker D.S. and Lieberman M.A. 1965 *Psychotherapy Through the Group Process*. Tavistock, London
8 Freeman R. 1987 The group dynamic. *Horizons*, July, 365–9
9 Lines K (ed.) 1973 *Greek Legends*. Faber and Faber, London
10 Cotterell A. 1989 *Myths and Legends*. Cassell Marshal Editions, London
11 Smail D. 1984 *Illusion and Reality – the Meaning of Anxiety* JM Dent, London

12 See for example Gardiner J. 1989 *The Anatomy of Supervision*. The Society for Research into Higher Education and the Open University Press, Milton Keynes

13 Rogers C. 1980 *A Way Of Being*. Houghton Mifflin, Boston

14 Hedley R. 1996 Individual education plans for GPs. *Education for General Practice*, **7**(1), 28–36

15 See for example Pitts J., Vincent S. and Percy D. (1996) The place of higher professional education in individual recertification. *Education for General Practice*, **7**(1), 8–15

16 Egan G. 1994 *The Skilled Helper*, 5th edn. Brooks/Cole Publishing, California

17 Brookfield S.D. 1996 *Understanding and Facilitating Adult Learning*. Open University Press, Milton Keynes

18 Marinker M. 1974 Medical education and human values. *Journal of the Royal College of General Practitioners*, **24**, 445–62

19 Heron J. 1986 *The Six Category Intervention Analysis Human Potential Research Project*, 2nd edn. University of Surrey, Guildford

20 Ibid

21 Kitchener K.S. 1986 The reflective judgement model. In *Adult Cognitive Development* (eds Mines R.A. and Kitchener K.S.). Praeger, New York

5

Using reflective practice for professional development

'The centipede was happy quite
Until the toad in fun
Said "pray which leg goes after which . . . "
And worked her mind to such a pitch,
She lay distracted in the ditch
Considering how to run'

(attributed to Mrs Edmund Craster, d. 1874, from
The Oxford Dictionary of Quotations, 2nd edn. 1953)

This chapter describes the process of introducing the concept of reflective practice to the mentors, using their local support groups as context. The concept of reflective practice, seen to be an important component of the mentoring relationship, was received with some ambivalence by mentors, as this chapter shows. The experience of the mentor groups is used to illustrate the conceptual framework of reflection, and some possible reasons for its mixed reception considered. The chapter concludes with some examples of how purposeful reflection brought to the mentor team further knowledge and skills for the mentor task.

Reflective practice

So far the work in the support groups had focused on developing the mentor's skills in establishing a purposeful and effective mentoring relationship with their mentee. The mentors legitimately expected that the support groups and plenary workshops would provide them with techniques and skills for managing the mentoring interviews – practical ways of becoming competent mentors. But this was only half the task. A further declared aim of the support groups was to attend to the mentor's own professional development, and herein lay a dilemma.

The first part of the previous chapter showed how, through their pre-occupation with structure, the mentors gave voice to their need to feel safe and in control of the mentoring process. As their work developed, and their confidence grew, many of the mentors balanced this with exploring the unknown, and sometimes the unspoken aspects of their mentee's agenda; in the process they were gradually learning to be more challenging, asking 'why' rather than telling 'how'. Similarly, in the developing interaction of the support groups, these were the mentors who carried through their developing style of working with their mentee into their work with their mentor–peers, using the experiential learning base of the group to explore the attitudes and beliefs that underpinned a mentor's actions, asking each other 'why' as well as 'how'.

Others expressed their caution about working in this way. These mentors, whilst they supported the validity of working in the more explorative and challenging way with mentees, showed a preference for working from the technical–rational perspective when working within the group with their peers. Like all doctors, they were used to staying firmly in control of the process of an interview and subsequently, in the support groups, they wished to stay firmly in control of themselves and the situation being presented. They sought solutions to complex problems of their mentor–peers, and tried to find 'proper answers' to resolve dilemmas for them. They more naturally used the logical, deductive thinking that stems from the dominant scientific paradigm of medicine. Yet, increasingly, there were occasions when, in different ways to their more adventurous colleagues, they owned their intuitive feeling that this familiar approach to problem-solving did not take them far enough down the road of holistic mentoring. One mentor voiced the intuition with startling clarity:

'sometimes I feel shackled . . . stuck with my own need for knowing and certainty'.

Within the mentor groups then there is a dilemma which Schon[1] sees as lying between rigour and relevance. Some mentors stood firmly on the high, hard ground of rigour, scientific certainty and 'knowing', whilst others descended fairly happily into the swampy ground, that messy, uncertain but important place, wherein lie issues and problems of crucial importance and relevance to the situation. The personal advantages and disadvantages to these stances are obvious – you are safer, more in control on the high ground, falling back on scientific reasoning to explain events, distanced from the mess and confusion of the swamps. Working in the swamps ensures relevance, working 'where it's at', yet constantly encountering uncertainty for which there is no body of knowledge to direct the outcome.

From my leadership role, the sense of threatened polarization was all too obvious, with the attendant risk of entrenching attitudes between the occupants of the high ground and the workers in the swamps, between 'thinkers' and 'feelers'. I needed to find a way out of this dilemma, an acceptable means of bridging the divide.

Now that the first intensity of getting started with their mentee had passed, the mentors became more aware of their own interaction with each other, and were poised to use each other as a source of feedback and learning. This in itself provided the first foothold in getting a purchase on the dilemma, and it enabled me to draw the mentor's attention to what was happening, using aspects of their interaction as evidence. In discussion, we could see more clearly that, whilst all mentors shared the vision of holistic mentoring, and its accompanying requirement for working in different components and at different levels, some mentors simply did not know how to unshackle themselves from known ways of addressing problems. They did not know where to start, beyond sensing that they needed to experience more of the difference for themselves, before trying it out with their mentees – a powerful reminder of Rogers' edict[2] that you can only take your client as far along the road as you have been yourself.

It seemed, therefore, that if this shared aspect of group life was to be tapped as the rich learning source it undoubtedly was, it had to be integrated into the learning process in a way which was accessible to our thinkers and technical–rationalists, so that sessions were not overtaken by our feeling swampies, carried away on the tide of their own discovery learning. To this end, I began to introduce into the support groups a format for presenting their work which borrowed from critical incident analysis (frequently used in general practice training) married up with methods of reflective practice.

For most of the mentor groups, finding the required starting point for reflective practice was a problem. To begin to engage in purposeful reflection requires the possession of attitudes which predispose us towards it, and, in the mentor teams, we did not all start from the same attitudinal place. An overarching prerequisite is a state of mind which says that it is not enough simply to 'know' – there has to be an accompanying desire to apply knowledge, and from that three attitudes are identified:

1. Open-mindedness: an ability to see a problem in new and different ways, contrary to one's own view
2. Wholeheartedness: involvement and engagement, interest and commitment
3. Responsibility – not only as a moral trait, but as a need to consider the consequences of action; part of one's intellectual resource.

Becoming a 'reflective practitioner' has become another throwaway phrase used lightly but extensively both in higher education and medicine. To bring about a well structured, purposeful reflection on experience is hard work; it goes beyond the sort of reflective daydreaming that most of us utilize when stuck in traffic jams, when we review the events of the working day. Indeed one of the advantages of attempting to travel the M25 is that one can fit in a review of one's entire life, but it is obvious that this is not exactly what is meant by reflection. Loughran,[3] for example, sees reflection as an infinitely more serious activity, much more of a deliberate act of inquiry into your thoughts and actions, a process which precedes the testing out of a reasoned response. This purposeful reflection is used as a means through which

'a thoughtful, reasoned response might be tested out',

widening perspectives on a problem (broadening knowledge), developing strategies for dealing with it (developing skills) and insights into behaviour (changing attitudes). This view of reflection was to become the cornerstone of the mentor group sessions, moving the work between Loughran's three reflective levels:

Anticipatory (what am I going to do in that situation)
Retrospective (what did I do in that situation), and
Contemporaneous (thinking on your feet).

The mentors already had their own experience of the power of reflection through their testing of the Reflective Cycle in the induction phase, and my intention was to build on this, extending the experience to encourage a move away from technical–rationality towards open-mindedness and wholeheartedness in going beyond the obvious. It did however bring us face to face again with the dilemma. Whilst many mentors – usually the feelers – when provided with a format for organizing the presentation of their work into a reflective framework – fell into reflective practice like proverbial ducks to water, others – usually the thinkers – struggled to find their way into a level of discussion and sharing which might be considered as purposeful reflection, preferring instead to skim the surface of their own experience, impatient with both the presentation format and the reflective process itself. The exasperated comment of one of the mentors during the discussion bore this out:

'we could reflect ourselves into a state of paralysis . . . we are in danger of analysing too much, thinking about it too long, instead of just getting on with it . . . doing it [mentoring].'

From my own position as the project leader, I saw purposeful reflection as an important part of the mentoring process, one of the aspects that took it beyond a mere conversation to a purposeful professional intervention. If, in the relative safety of their peer group, mentors themselves were unable to enter into a process of purposeful reflection on their work, what was the likelihood that they could use their mentor interviews as an opportunity to offer this different experience to their mentees?

It was clear that some mentors were being urged to go places they did not want to go, for serious reflection is a process that does not always lead to comfortable outcomes, can undermine certainty and might thereby erode a necessary image of themselves as managing their mentor role adequately.

It was comforting to find parallels of the problem in the development of reflective practice in teacher education. Here, students in teacher training programmes are preoccupied with learning how to become a teacher, whilst their educators are preoccupied with finding ways of relating to their students to enable this to happen. I identified with this – I felt the mentors were preoccupied with how to become an effective mentor, whilst I was preoccupied with finding ways of facilitating that learning.

I tried to define the difference between the mentors who had taken to the reflective waters, adopting a questioning, reflective attitude to their own work, and those who stood back from this, staying on the margins of reflecting on experience. A clue was provided in the work of Entwhistle[4] who demonstrated that, as people perceive and process information in qualitatively different ways, teachers need to know more about how their students understand and use their experience if they are to develop effective teaching methods.

In his later work[5] he urged that teachers needed to take account of the range of learning styles of their students, and be familiar with their own, as these were likely to be reflected in their teaching. Without these insights,

'the style of teaching might be personally satisfying to the teacher, but would impose on other students an alien way of learning.'[6]

This seemed to exactly mirror our dilemma. For some group members, my attempt to introduce a more structured reflection format was an alien way of going about things. In his learning style inventory, Kolb[7] drew from Jungian concepts when he implied that all of us have dominant learning functions – preferred learning styles. The mentor support groups and the developmental workshops were designed to encourage the mentors to move away from preferred learning styles and dominant functions, to engage in the discovery of the more dormant aspects of themselves. Working in this way would (it was hypothesized) extend their ability to work flexibly with their mentees, to use all the different aspects of their own personality, and in the process, discover these for themselves. This learning could then be further applied to personal and professional development, and become part of the process of self-actualization and role-fulfilment.

So much for the learner's part in all this. But Kolb is quick to make the link between preferred learning styles and teaching styles, showing how the relationship between the teacher's preferred learning styles influences their preferred teaching stance. He alerts teachers to be equally aware of their own learning style, and that of their students, so that the teacher can develop a range of teaching styles which allows them to respond flexibly to the differing needs of their students.

Talking with mentors about my own role as leader, facilitator, and at times teacher, showed how my own preferred teaching style was at odds with some of the mentors, and at times alienated them from the core content, or main message of a group session. Bringing this into the open moved the groups markedly closer together, and from this sense of increased trust and acceptance, we were able to consider the part that personality plays in the development of a professional role.

Preferred learning styles, indeed any preference for conducting a particular role, is rooted in our basic personality type; for example Jung[8] saw four basic function types which he perceived as a four point axis (Figure 5.1).

In the centre of the four functions is the ego, the source of energetic willpower, the transforming process. Jung used his typology not to put people into boxes, labelling them as 'thinkers' or 'feelers', but as an organizing principle, to conceptualize dominant 'superior' functions, which, when engaged obliterate the opposite 'inferior' functions. In the case of the thinking type, the ego's energy is directed towards thinking, and thinking becomes the dominant or superior function, with feeling below it as the inferior function, simply because, as Jung says:

'when you think, you must exclude feeling, just as when you feel, you must exclude thinking. If you are thinking, leave feeling and feeling values alone, because feeling is most upsetting to your thoughts. On the other hand, people who go by feeling values leave thinking well alone, and they are right to do so, because these two different functions contradict each other . . . an individual cannot have the two opposites in the same degree of perfection at the same time' (pp. 16–17).

Whilst recognizing that at different times in one's life one of the polarities is dominant – for example, the cognitive, thinking domain would be uppermost when pursuing a course of study, with the intuitive domain being less dominant, Jung more strongly emphasizes the need for fluidity, to be able to move around the axis and experience all four polarities at

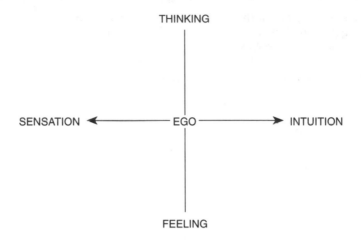

Figure 5.1 Jungian model of four basic function types

different times, as a prerequisite for personal development; another step in the road towards 'wholeness' and self fulfilment.

In the mentor teams, many of the mentors whose dominant functions were intuitive, or feeling, naturally found reflective practice more to their liking; these were the ones with additional training in counselling, stress management, and alternative medicine. The nature of this additional learning suggested that these mentors had been exposed to ways of processing information and experience which was outside of traditional methods of medical training. Their previous, familiar learning styles had already undergone a challenge, and consequently their axis had been moved around, and they appeared more flexible and exploratory than their colleagues, more at home with different aspects of themselves. Indeed, when interviewing one mentor, there was evidence that medical training and subsequent practice can in itself serve to lock the axis into an immovable position in which the doctor senses the presence of other, dormant functions but cannot find a way of releasing them:

'I felt enormous discomfort about medicine as it had been taught, and medicine as we were 'expected' to practise it. I felt increasingly uncomfortable about practising this way, and living this way, and I got to the point of wondering – do I actually want to go on being a doctor at all . . . But . . . there were lots of pressures on me . . . the reality it was I had to stay – but if I had to stay I would do it differently, and I stayed and did it absolutely differently . . . It wore me out to start with but now I have got a much better sense of when I have to be one kind of doctor and when I can be another, and I can be many, many different kinds of doctor . . . this is what connects me with mentoring. I have a sense of the different aspects of myself.'

In discussing with the mentor team the issue of learning styles, and the way in which shared learning can lead to discovery of different parts of the self, some mentors reflected on their past experience of being members of Balint groups. Balint[9] is a deserving if surprising guru of general practice;

surprising in that, as early as the 1950s, he held firmly to the psychological component of illness, in the face of the intransigence of scientifically-based medicine. His pioneering concept of the centrality of the doctor/patient relationship, with the doctor himself as the most powerful drug on offer to the patient, was achieved through a series of reflective groups – Balint groups. The nature of these groups meant that members came away with an experience of deeply searching, reflection-on-action which was, by anecdotal account, of such a profound nature that participants either left the group, or stayed with it and changed the whole basis of their practice and beliefs.

Other mentors in the teams had experienced Balint groups, and left swiftly, knowing that this style was not for them. Sharing these different experiences highlighted the importance of addressing the disparity in preferred learning styles, of continually monitoring the learning process of the mentor groups, and making sure that they were useful events to all participants.

Ownership

One of the most positive aspects of general practitioners' need to be in control of their learning is that, once a problem is identified in a learning group, there is tremendous positive force to set about resolving it, and it was the same in the mentor groups. Identifying the potential divide between thinkers and feelers, showing how it found its way into the group's interaction, gave permission for mentors to be honest about their different learning styles, and not feel they had to conform to an imposed style. Once this was acknowledged, polarities lessened – the intuitive feelers dug out their rational, logistical thinking modes, and the thinking sensors tested out intuition and feeling.

Two further important shifts then occurred in the mentoring scheme. Firstly, the overt recognition of the mix of learning styles meant that the mentors quickly moved into learning from each other, and gradually but progressively the learning process was led, verbalized and conducted by the mentors themselves – they began to take over the leadership and ownership of their support groups, to sustain their action. Alongside this came the second shift, when, through the closer working with each other, they discovered the transformative power of learning and leadership. They themselves took on the task of bridging the potential disparity of learning styles, and produced meaningful learning for each other at quite challenging levels. This extract from my notes of a group session provides a snapshot of how they achieved this:

H follows on [from a previous discussion] and presents us with her reflection on her actions in a recent mentoring session, describing the process of the mentoring interview in a lively and engaged way. She finishes her reflection with saying, 'you know . . . C [the mentee] will never stick general practice.'

An astonished silence, but then the group is quick to explore this assumptive behaviour. Firmly but gently, the mentor's own beliefs are explored to see where this assumption came from, and to consider other experiences of 'hunches' that might become untested assumptions, and whether hunches have a place in mentoring relationships. It is a very wide-ranging discussion, using lots of psychological and sociological frameworks, until eventually with some exasperation B, another mentor, says, 'but my mentees need practical help'. She reflects on her inner responses and subsequent action when, at one stage in the mentoring interview, the mentee had asked, 'what do you think I should do?'

This is taken up by the group, largely in terms of supporting mentees to make their own decision. They discuss how they perceive the role of the mentor as one which goes beyond that of offering peer support, to one which provided some challenge which helps the mentees move forward in their thinking – 'after all, we wouldn't be sitting here unless we had that extra bit to offer . . . that other dimension'. I commented generally that mentees might be uncomfortable with this unfamiliar 'other' dimension, and the freedom of exploration that mentoring provides.

After a pause, B [the mentor with the practical mentee] says hesitantly that she herself is concerned that she might miss possible other dimensions in her mentoring. Example? 'well . . . being a 'practical' person . . . do I miss the mentee's inner agenda?' Being a practical person, she sees herself more easily giving practical advice, but is now concerned that in this, she is out of step with the other mentors, who seem to her to be working at 'more depth'. The group discusses the perennial anxiety for mentors – 'is it me or is it them?' – does the mentee only want practical, straightforward advice, or am I unable to move the discussion into another level where the inner agenda might be revealed? The group works with B to relate this to her experience with her mentee, saying, in effect, that it is not either/or – but perhaps it can be both – practical advice, and exploratory, and reflective. B thinks on this and then says she finds her mentee 'hard to get to know'. Is it me – or him? The group points out that as the mentee is one of 14 doctors in a multi-group practice perhaps he is unused to being 'known', and doesn't quite know how to reveal more of himself. Finally, A [mentor and ex-Balint member] and I between us venture that it is a challenge to mentors to become known also to themselves.

There is appreciative recognition from the group that this is the first time that B has voiced her concerns; in fact they are so dead keen to help her they keep falling over themselves to speak. And then H tells B that she has found her contribution to the discussion very helpful. 'Yes,' I say, 'but why?' H says because she is such a 'feely' person she feels she needs some of B's practicality. B laughs and says she envies H her ability to be intuitive, and 'feely'. 'Right then,' says A, 'you two can get together and do some swapping around . . .

The climate of this working session enabled preferred ways of working as a mentor to be shared, and some attempts made to begin shifting the axis around to incorporate other, less familiar responses. The mentors worked at reflection wholeheartedly, and sought open-mindedness.

Confrontation

Coming to terms with the reality of reflective practice included trying out for ourselves Schon's[10] reflection *on* action – how the mentors reviewed and analysed their actions when they thought back over their work – and at times their 'knowing *in* action', or unpacking the process of 'thinking on your feet'. Through this process we came to see that, although the mentor groups were using reflective pathways, they were in fact reconstructing Schon's model of reflection. Using the structured format for

reflection moved the teams away from Schon's privatized notion of reflection, towards employing it in an open and communal way. In *sharing* with
each other their individual reflections on their different ways of perceiving
and framing the mentee's problems, and their planned and unplanned
responses to events in the mentoring session, each mentor's practice
became public. This aspect of going public lies at the heart of criticisms
about Schon's framework. He appears to see reflection as a personal and
private task, yet it is only through making private reflections accessible
to others, and placing them in the public domain so that they can be
talked about and understood more widely, that practice can be developed
and, when necessary, improved.*

However, as was said earlier, such public reflection is not always comfortable, and it heightens feelings of vulnerability. At times we had to
confront that vulnerability and, when doing so, made overt a further continuing theme of mentoring, that of confrontation. Mentors wanted to
consider more carefully the appropriate use of themselves in confronting
difficult areas in the mentoring process, and construction confrontation
was worked with at two levels. At one level, confrontation was seen as
an organizational issue related to managing the process of the mentoring
session; as is seen here, when a mentor describes to his group his feelings
about a recent meeting with his mentee:

'I sat there thinking . . . I've lost control of this session . . . it's all over the shop . . .
we are wasting time here . . . Then I suddenly found myself saying so; I actually
said out loud, "It might just be me . . . but I am feeling that I am losing the
thread of this . . . we seem to be casting around a bit . . . would it be useful to
go back to the partnership agreement . . . , because I sensed you felt angry
about that at the time . . . "'

With his group, this mentor shared his feeling of vulnerability, in losing
control, but also showed how, despite this, he had used his own feelings
to make an offer and strike out for another shore. This prompted discussion amongst the mentors of their own experiences of feeling vulnerable
with their peers, of being seen as less than all-coping, and all-knowing.
This discussion also had wider echoes and introduced the second aspect
of confrontation, which goes beyond using it to manage the organizational
process of the mentoring session, to managing a confrontation with individuals about their own behaviours and attitudes in described events.

Learning to confront, to challenge the behaviour and responses of
others without destroying them or yourself in the process, became a recur-
rent theme in both teams. This is a difficult skill for anyone to develop,
whatever the context of their work, but for general practice mentors it
was even harder, for they themselves carried the legacies of negative learning described earlier in the chapter. This meant that their own experience
of being confronted was usually destructive, it being an intervention aimed
at belittling, or attacking; like their mentees, they had little experience of
receiving positive feedback during their professional lives with which to

*I am grateful to Professor John Elliott for his insight and help in illuminating the complex-
ities of reflective practice.

balance the negative experience against. So the mentors had little security from which to move out on this one, for although they knew about confronting patients, the power base of the consultation was very different from the equal relationship with their peer-mentee. And when I, as their group leader, confronted them with the need to hold up the mirror and show the mentee that aspect of themselves which, in their behaviours and responses, contributed to the very situation that they so bitterly complained of, there was a general air of discomfort, as these field notes show:

G [the mentor] describes his struggle to try to help his mentee 'get in touch' with the acerbic, at times aggressive, part of her nature. Although the mentee unhappily relates the arguments she has at work with the practice manager, and how miserable these make her, she seems unable to see that if she speaks to her colleagues in the way that she at times speaks to the mentor, particularly when making appointments on the phone, it is not surprising that the practice manager acts defensively. The mentor feels uneasily that it goes further than the practice manager; the mentee had told him recently that all the other partners get cups of tea brought to them in their surgery to sustain them, but J [the mentee] never does . . . ! Lots of strategies for 'wrapping up' the message are discussed. I ask, 'why do we have to give coded messages?' Surely the mentee gets enough of those from her colleagues in the practice, and clearly they have not been heard. Could the mentor not use his own experience to feed back to the mentee that he has experienced her at times as being somewhat aggressive, and has often been puzzled by her response; could they explore this together and then see if any of that related to the situation in the practice? All the group shift around; someone sighs impatiently [she's off again]. 'It sounds a bit dangerous', says someone. 'Why?' 'You might upset the mentee, she might feel criticized, it would end the relationship, etc. etc.' 'But,' I say, 'is the mentee that fragile? I am doing something similar with all of you now – confronting you with your resistance to confrontation, as it were. Is this likely to end our relationship?' Dead silence. I try and explain (not very coherently) the difference between criticizing, scoring points, attacking, and using your own experience with a person to give them a starting point to explore the uncomfortable bits of themselves. After a heavy pause, N says that he thinks that perhaps that's what the mentee is asking for; in a way, she wants to know why she is treated differently. I restrain myself from hugging him, and instead reinforce the value of confronting, not to destroy, but to try to unpack the complicated process of interpersonal communication. The atmosphere changes; we all breathe more easily.

In this glimpse of leadership life as lived in the mentor support group is the interaction of a confronting leader, the facilitator, who makes life uncomfortable. Brookfield again:[11]

'the teacher of adults, then, is not always engaged in a warm and wholly satisfying attempt to assist adults in their innate drive to achieve self-actualisation. Analysing assumptions, challenging previously accepted and internalised values, considering the validity of alternative behaviours . . . all these acts are at times uncomfortable, and all involve pain. The outcome of these activities may be a more satisfactory level of self-insight, but these experiences may induce . . . feelings of insecurity' (p.125).

In the example of my own leadership problem, as at other times, I was able to use my own relationship with the mentors, and liken it to their relationship with their mentee. In Mattinson's[12] little book about the process of reflection in casework supervision, she shows how often the processes at work between the helper and client (in our context mentor and the mentee) are often reflected in the relationship between the worker and their supervisor (the mentor and myself and the group as supervisor). Whilst this is an uncomfortable reflection, she says, it is too good to miss – actively using it and reflecting it back powerfully de-mists the mirror.

When the mentee acts with (apparently) unnecessary aggression, she not unnaturally arouses a defensive response in her mentor. Like the mentee's colleagues, he too wanted to withdraw; he didn't want to make her a cup of tea either. When I as 'supervisor' confronted these feelings, he and his group at first became defensive, thinking me dangerous, and they wanted to withdraw. But we managed to hang in there, and when we came out the other side, I could offer my own confrontation with the group as one example of how to go about it.

Overall though, in establishing a working relationship with the mentor teams, challenge was balanced in equal measure with support. Finding opportunities to give positive feedback to mentors was not difficult, for the professional and conscientious way in which they set about developing their skills and knowledge was extraordinary, earning not only my admiration, but also the appreciation of those who worked with the mentor teams more occasionally as external resources in developmental workshops.

As the project moved out from its implementation phase, and settled into becoming an ongoing regional scheme, funded by the Postgraduate Dean, there was an increasing sense of establishment. The mentors developed confidence in their strengths, and they became much clearer about the requirements of their task. They put their developing experience to good use, presenting their work in various public arenas, writing about their experiences of being a mentor, and taking many initiatives which would publicize their availability to other potential mentors. All of this went beyond the bounds of simply practising the task of mentoring, but mentors showed their continuing commitment to the vision by giving their additional time freely and enthusiastically. They began the process of reviewing and re-defining the holistic model, for example, rewriting some of the frameworks for recording mentoring sessions, and looking again at the way in which their work was evaluated by their mentees.

Why is all this being reported here you ask? Not because it imparts a happy glow necessarily, although of course it does, but because it leads on to another important part of the story. The mentors had served their apprenticeship and, as the volume of work developed and other skills and knowledge were drawn in, they had completed their time as journeymen and women. In doing all these things and more, the mentor teams began to make mentoring their own project and identify with the holistic model as a relevant part of general practice work. They had discovered the reality of acting as a mentor: that they did not need enormous stockpiles of answers and infinite wisdom, but instead the capacity of reflective judgement[13] which works outside the boundaries of certain knowledge, allowing you to give up the need to 'know' in favour of exploring the reason why. They had spread their wings over some ravines, and found that men and women could cross safely to the other side.

Through the learning which came from the privileged experience of working with their mentees, and their shared experience in the mentor support groups, the mentors began to see their potential as change agents in their profession. They saw what mentoring could become in their hands. They were becoming masters of their own craft, so that I took a step back from the leadership role, and they took the project on. Naturally then, it is the mentors who tell the next part of the story.

References

1   Schon D. 1983 *The Reflective Practitioner – How Professionals Think in Action*. Basic Books
2   Rogers C.R. 1980 *A Way of Being*. Houghton Mifflin, Boston MA
3   Loughran J. 1996 *Developing Reflective Practice*. Falmer Press, London
4   Entwhistle N.J. 1981 *Styles of Learning and Teaching*. Wiley, London
5   Entwhistle N.J. 1991 Cognitive style and learning. In *The Foundations of Students' Learning* (ed. Marjoribanks K.) Pergamon, Oxford
6   Ibid pp. 144–5
7   Kolb D. 1984 *Experiential Learning*. Englewood Cliffs, New York NJ
8   C.G. Jung 1968 *Analytical Psychology – its Theory and Practice*. Routledge and Kegan Paul, London
9   Balint M. 1994 (reprinted) *The Doctor, His Patient, and the Illness*. Churchill Livingstone
10 Ibid
11 Ibid
12 Mattinson J. 1975 *The Reflection Process in Casework Supervision*. Institute of Marital Studies, Tavistock Institute of Human Relations, London
13 Kitchener K.S. 1986 The reflective judgement model. In *Adult Cognitive Development* (eds Mines R.A. and Kitchener K.S.) Praeger, New York

6

The mentor's and the mentee's tale

This chapter begins with some thoughts on the necessary personal qualities of a mentor, and is followed by a personal account of mentoring from two practising mentors. The voices of four mentees then tell something of their experience of being mentored.

It is around this stage of telling a story that the questions gathering in the minds of the listeners erupt as the tale unfolds. The storyteller is interrupted by those who are impatient with the actions of the characters and needs to advise them how best to proceed, or those wanting to know if there is a happy ending to come. Interruptions like these are reassuring; they indicate an audience engaged with the tale, who can identify with the heroes and heroines, whilst recognizing in themselves the capacity to act as the wicked witch, or become the Accursed One.

For those such readers, amongst the questions raised by previous chapters might be: What kind of people become mentors? Can I identify with them? Are they ordinary practitioners and people, or do they possess exceptional qualities that marks them out as mentors? And what of their mentees – are they any different from me? What made them seek out a mentor in the first place – are they glad they did, or might they now have regrets?

In this chapter, through their writing, the voices of two practitioners who became mentors are heard, both of whom tell us something about their motivation to take on the job, and perhaps, through their writing, show something of their personal qualities that make them effective mentors.

Mentor types

How 'typical' are these two mentors of mentors overall? In the first year of the mentor project, and later, as the project work developed, I carried out some semi-structured interviews with mentors. Amongst the many questions I wanted to discover answers to was whether members of this self-selected mentor team conformed to any stereotypes. Were there any common motivating factors for taking on the task and, if so, were these the manifestations of common attributes which made it more (or less) likely that someone would 'make a good mentor'? It was an ambitious task, and one early outcome of it was to realize exactly why protagonists in the mentoring field, all far more worthy and experienced than I, had fudged the issue of requisite mentor qualities. Mentoring relationships are in themselves both unique and complex, and as such confound attempts to make precise and objective statements about the particular qualities required by the mentor beyond those that have previously been discussed, all of which come under the general heading of being 'facilitating' or 'enabling'.

Talking at some depth with mentors about their motivation showed that they had in common a concern for the stressed state of their profession, and the effects that this turbulent working climate had on general practitioners. But then many doctors shared that sense of concern, and were not motivated to try actively to change it. Equally, as was seen in the introductory workshops, and in subsequent support groups, not all mentors displayed consistent qualities that marked them out as the angels that Allah intended to help men, as 'good' mentor material.

Motivation

Reflecting on those early interviews, and adding in more understanding and knowledge of their content as the mentor scheme developed, it seemed that some mentors were in part prompted into action by their own remembered experience of being cared for in mentor-type relationships. For example, one mentor talked with warm affection of the games mistress at her boarding school, who had noticed her miserable homesickness, and taken time to talk sympathetically about this, in the process encouraging and supporting a mastery of school life which the mentor now saw had laid the foundation for a positive mastery of life itself. Another had experienced a mentor-type relationship in his Young Principals group, at a time when he felt incredibly angry that, after years of training, he should feel so inexperienced and inept when finally becoming a principal in practice. These and other examples were not uppermost in the minds of the mentors as motivating factors when they offered themselves for the task, but were recalled easily and vividly in the interview, and perhaps served as an unconscious, but encouraging factor in their decision to take on the role.

Attributes

Those practitioners who decided to join the mentor scheme as mentors were self selected, and the initial training purposefully did not attempt to prescribe attributes necessary for the task. Whilst I have never believed that just anybody can 'do' mentoring, neither do I believe that it is immediately obvious as to who should do it. Chapter 2 shows how the interpretations of the mentor's role can vary with the context of their work, and range from teacher, coach and adviser, to guide, counsellor and inspirer. Whilst the holistic model of mentoring implied qualities in a mentor which enabled them to enter into a voyage of discovery with their mentee, an enabling function which went beyond a mechanized view of an educational mentor, the lack of any clear knowledge base of mentoring in general practice made a precise definition of mentor attributes presumptuous. But, as our mentoring work has developed, and consequently our knowledge base grown, the question of mentor attributes has become more focused on selecting mentors who appear likely to possess the *potential* to develop a range of skills which move along the pole of facilitating personal journeys at one end, and providing pragmatic advice at the other, rather than only seeking those who obviously display these abilities.

When and where are the seeds of such mentor-potential sown? Do they come from outside, via our encounters with others, so that if we ourselves experience people who listen to us, give us their attention, support and encourage us in a particular life event, or coach us to perform a role adequately, we are more likely to develop similar qualities which we can draw upon to use elsewhere when the opportunity presents itself? Or does the ability to pay genuine attention and concern to the agenda of others, without seeking direct or obvious profit to oneself, come not from our outside experience of others, but from inside, within the self? At the heart of the concept of the 'wounded healer' is the belief that when the doctor confronts his or her own experience of personal dishevelment, and lets the mask of infallibility fall, they gain immeasurably from the encounter. Carl Jung was emphatic that only the wounded physician heals, for when doctors have the experience of becoming a patient themselves, they develop a closer affinity with the common humanity of illness, often to the great benefit of their patients.

In the two following accounts, Neil Munro and Peter Harborow share their experience of becoming mentors, and their views on the process of a mentoring relationship. Their writing displays their different personalities, so that these personal stories show something of the complexity of questions about mentor qualities. At times they offer answers to some of the questions, but most of all they offer readers insights from which to formulate their own thoughts about these, and other mentor matters.

On becoming a mentor

Neil Munro

'A fortuitous relationship that fosters an adult's development'[1]

Motivation

History is peppered with examples of famous mentoring relationships. Freud and Jung, Haydn and Beethoven and Socrates and Plato benefited from powerful 'emotional interactions between an older and younger person, in which the older member is trusted, loving and experienced in the guidance of the younger.'[2] Despite the 'definition quagmire'[3] surrounding mentoring, its role in professional and personal development continues to attract my own, and others' considerable interest. In the opening chapter, the point was made that interest in mentoring in general practice coincided with a period of turbulent change. I look back and see that the 1990s heralded significant changes for general practice within the National Health Service. Imposition of a new contract for family doctors increased emphasis on financial control and cost-effectiveness. Additionally, governmental fuelling of patient expectation considerably increased the strain on individual practitioners already perceiving themselves to be under excessive pressure in their working environment. In its report to the Doctors' and Dentists' Review Body, the British Medical

Association pointed to a 20% national decline in the number of general practice registrars between 1986 and 1996.[4] The recognition that occupational stress may be contributing to the decline in general practice as a preferred career option among medical graduates has reinforced the belief among many practitioners and educators, one which I share, that a system of professional support is urgently needed in family medicine.[5]

The question of whether general practice mentors might promote individual doctors' sense of well being, as well as enabling on-going professional development, formed the basis of a feasibility study into effective mentoring in general practice within South Thames (West) Region.[6] I first became aware of this initiative in late 1994. A letter from the offices of the Postgraduate Dean invited general practitioners, interested in participating in the research, to a workshop on initial skills for mentors. The aims of the workshop were fourfold:

> To establish a knowledge base of the mentoring task
> To place the work of GP mentors in the wider context of professional mentoring
> To provide participants with initial, relevant training in mentor skills
> To offer a forum for development of ideas and skills in mentoring.

Mentors have long existed in commercial and educational environments but had only recently entered the arena of professions such as medicine. The concept that mentoring could invigorate and revitalize the working and private lives of family doctors offered a temptingly optimistic alternative to the depressingly negative picture of contemporary general practice so frequently portrayed in the medical press.

Initiation

Only those responding to the first letter from the research team attended the initial workshop. This self-selected group of potential mentors demonstrated at least some commitment to mentoring simply by taking time out of their practices. Some, but not all, had educational backgrounds. Most were experienced general practitioners. None reported previous mentoring encounters in any formal sense but some had had formative moments of self-reflection during their professional careers.

My true awakening to the empowering potential of mentoring relationships occurred during that first workshop. After an overview of mentoring models, including specifically the holistic model to be used in the study, we were split into pairs and asked to mentor one another in turn. For probably the first time in my adult life, I was given ample space to talk about aspects of my own professional development. I chose 'future plans' as the segment of the reflective cycle to explore, initially imagining it a 'safe' area to share with my workshop partner, whom I had not previously met. To my surprise I soon became enmeshed in quite profound analysis of both my professional and personal aspirations and emerged with a plan for the next few years. Those 20 minutes of permitted self-reflection significantly influenced my career path and instilled a feeling of direction and control over my own life I had not felt for some time. The beneficent nature of fortuitous relationships became firmly cemented in my mind.

This initial experience of mentoring reinforced my belief that the process is one few clinicians should miss. The opportunity to consider one's position and future in the company of a non-judgmental and well disposed peer seemed new and exciting. It broke with the subservience and overt patronage so familiar in professional medical relationships and provided an environment in which success and failure might be explored without risk of ridicule or career disadvantage. The ability of the mentor to set aside personal agendas and devote time solely to the mentee is crucial to success within a mentoring relationship. During this first encounter I had gained a sense of the 'specialness' that has characterized mentoring in other occupational fields. Whilst somewhat reticent about exploring personal as opposed to professional issues within a mentoring encounter I became acutely aware of the potential the process had to facilitate professional development.

Taking up the mentor role

In contrast to my first experience as a mentee in the workshop, I found the role of mentor more difficult to immediately assimilate. Although the need for experience and empathy seemed self-evident, the further requirements of a mentor cited in the literature showed why developing a mentor identity would take time. Perkoff[7] cited 'interactive charisma' as an important trait in a successful mentor and added that 'neither a flat affect nor a dull mind is conducive to good mentoring'. Levinson[8] included roles such as teacher, sponsor, counsellor, developer of skills and intellect, host, guide and exemplar as well as dream facilitator in his taxonomy of mentor characteristics. Hagerty[9] emphasized the need for mentors to recognize when to 'stand back and allow a mentee to develop in autonomous ways'. Precisely how any of us could match up to the myriad of personal characteristics deemed essential or desirable in good mentors seemed at times quite unclear. This was all the more difficult since many of the recognized attributes were not only difficult to define but almost impossible to measure.

Other than demonstrating a willingness to give mentees undivided attention and enabling them to determine the content and agenda of the mentoring sessions, general practice mentors involved in the project were not required to provide objective evidence of skill for the task in hand. There is, however, an understanding that in the support groups mentors feed back to the scheme leader, and to their mentor peers, the themes that come through their mentoring encounters. This feedback has two main purposes. It provides some tangible evidence of the content and style of mentoring encounters to the team, as a basis for our learning, as well as confirming themes in the evaluation data which were so essential to our work when it was a research project, and subsequently as it continues to develop as a regional scheme. The monitoring of mentoring, albeit by very informal means, was thus built into the support structure from the very beginning.

Some concerns were expressed about confidentiality and the type of information to be recorded; if it were to be seen by those not directly involved in the mentoring relationship, particularly as our mentees trusted our ability to keep their disclosures to ourselves. The group decided, after some discussion, that the mentor and mentee could jointly undertake to record themes and key issues in a record of a mentor interview, but that the personal details of the mentee would not be returned on any of the forms. In addition to the record kept of the mentor session, and in order to assess the quality of their experiences, mentees were asked to comment on their mentoring encounters using 6-monthly review forms as well as exit questionnaires when leaving the scheme. This system remains broadly intact today.

The experience of becoming a mentor

The importance of the first meeting with a new mentee was emphasized during the initial workshop. Armed with our folders containing the developmental cycle and a list of prompting questions designed to 'set the ball rolling' we returned to our practices to await a call. Before I had time to reconsider precisely what I was getting myself involved in the 'call' arrived. I made contact with the doctor concerned and arranged to meet him the following week. Our meeting was very amicable and we covered a far wider range of areas than I had thought likely, in 2 hours. During the session he returned several times to seek clarification of precisely what mentoring was intended to achieve. I was never certain that I really answered that question. Despite some uncertainty about what was to be achieved by mentoring he was keen to meet again. Thus, it seems, the elusiveness of a precise definition of mentoring does not seem to diminish its attractiveness as a supportive intervention.

We met on a number of subsequent occasions over an 18-month period. The difficulties within his practice related to workload, funding of premises and on-call arrangements. In addition he was keen to extend his educational experience. We looked at this area through a learning contract. It was not easy to see whether things improved for him during the mentoring period. The process may have offered him the opportunity to reflect on the changing events that impinged on his working and private life. It may also have given give him a chance to gain a sense of perspective and provided a climate in which he could freely express his frustrations and ambitions.

Our meetings came to an end naturally. There was some difficulty keeping to prearranged times in very busy schedules. Most mentoring takes place in practitioners' 'spare' time. There is no provision for protected mentoring time within the terms of service for general practitioners in England and Wales. I learned early on to ask mentees whether they really wanted to meet again. Family doctors have to be particularly adept at time management and remain aware that many people want their undivided attention besides the patients whom they serve. I was very conscious of the preciousness of time we were using for mentoring not only from the mentee's point of view but from that of my own family. As I took on more mentees I realized that the pressures on my time might influence my ability to focus entirely on the mentee's agenda and took steps to limit the number I was seeing at any one time to three.

The issue of ending has never been a particularly easy one. Besides omitting to ask mentees explicitly whether they wanted to continue I occasionally failed to pick up the non-verbal cues indicating that 'winding up' would be appropriate. As the project progressed, and funding came from the offices of the Postgraduate Dean rather than a research grant, clear criteria have been developed that include a formal review of the mentoring process by both mentor and mentee after four meetings. If there is a need to continue, the focus of continuing work can be restated. Whilst primarily intended as a means of financial control this has had the effect, beneficial in my view, of introducing systematic appraisal into the regional mentoring system.

Having broken the ice with a male mentee slightly older than myself, my next two mentees were female. Although different in age their agendas were remarkably similar. Both were keen to develop in their practices and were committed to family medicine. One was specifically seeking support whilst sitting a higher professional examination. Both had significant relationship problems with a male partner in their practices and had already been to considerable lengths to improve matters. They were distressed by their situations and looking to re-establish sound perspectives. It was impossible not to be moved by their accounts. I was impressed at the skill and courage shown in dealing with the bullying and intimidating behaviour of their male counterparts.

I often wondered whether these antagonistic partners had ever imagined how they came across to others. I formulated the image of a 'pathological' partner. Immersed in their own agendas and incapable of responding to the needs of others, pathological partners appeared ubiquitous. Most practices seemed to have one. Whilst there are always two sides to a story and each of us, in certain circumstances, is capable of reprehensible behaviour towards one another, it was the repeated and persistent insensitivity of these doctors that was remarkable. Did these 'pathological' partners have any notion of the distress they caused? Were they capable of showing compassion and sensitivity towards those with whom they worked or did they simply not care? Would they themselves benefit from mentoring? Would the process help them see how the way they behaved caused so much unhappiness among others?

The possibility of attitudes changing through mentoring has been researched within teaching. In their study of formal mentoring programmes for elementary teachers Klug and Salzman[10] found improvements in attitude to work among mentored teachers. It is difficult to measure attitudinal change – I can say that I have seen changes in the attitudes of my mentees, and I know that some of my own attitudes have changed through the experience of becoming a mentor. If these attitudinal improvements could be repeated within mentoring programmes in medicine, the potential for improving the working conditions of large numbers of doctors would be enormous.

Personally, I find the issue interesting of whether matching mentor and mentee gender influences the outcome of mentoring, although I have worked equally comfortably with men and women. In my experience, the difference between mentoring male and female mentees is more to do with setting of boundaries rather than type of issues raised. The holistic model of mentoring allows free exploration of its three component elements: education, personal support and professional development.[11] Inevitably personal elements of our lives impinge, at times adversely, on our ability to develop professionally. On occasions mentoring can touch on areas of enormous sensitivity in an individual's personal life. The ensuing catharsis is often helpful but can take both mentor and mentee by surprise. If I sensed that discussion was straying into unexpected territory I would ask my mentee if she wanted to go any further. As in consultations with patients of the opposite sex there may be times when it can be very difficult, especially for a female mentee, to fully share her concerns with a male mentor. In addition I sometimes felt uncertain just how far some personal issues could be explored within the context of mentoring. The uniqueness of a mentoring relationship sets it apart from friendship, partnership or marriage in all aspects apart from its inherent intimacy.

In the event any real anxieties I had about relating to members of the opposite sex melted away as the relationships developed. I found that the mentees were more than capable of setting their own agendas and we would cross more boundaries as time went on.

There were odd times when I had to set the boundaries with mentees irrespective of their sex. I was asked to provide personal medical advice on occasions. Although happy to talk in general terms about aspects of medicine I was uneasy with a role of surrogate general practitioner. Most mentees were acutely aware of how the relationship between mentor and mentee differed from professional relationships in daily practice and rarely took on the role of a patient. In turn I tried consciously to behave as a mentor and not a doctor. I was not always successful. Finding a line between compassionate support for someone having a very difficult time and suggesting treatment for an underlying depression was problematic. Remaining totally medically detached seemed quite unnatural.

Mentoring is not solely about looking at people's problems. Many mentees were managing their lives reasonably well but were looking to improve things further. Even those seemingly overwhelmed by conflict or differences in their practices wanted to seek a way forward and explore their futures. The pursuit of happiness is a universal activity and the yearning for it is no less evident among general practitioners than among other members of society. Mentoring offers the opportunity for doctors to look at where they are now and where they wish to be in years ahead. It enables more precise definition of current obstacles to career progression. In addition the process can help individuals become consciously aware of their innermost aspirations. Levinson's[12] definition of the mentor as a 'dream facilitator' closely embodies this concept. Most of us have experienced formative moments when a remark, often made quite casually, has encouraged us to follow a certain path. If mentoring could summon these moments of enlightenment its potential to improve the quality of lives would be considerable.

Francis[13] describes a set of career drivers that we all possess to differing extents. These include attributes such as power and influence, material reward, expertise, security, status, creativity, affiliation, autonomy and the search for meaning. He emphasizes the need for people to maintain at least some control over the direction of their lives and argues that by understanding how we are motivated we are more likely to fulfil our ambitions. The elucidation of career drivers among mentees was identified by many mentees to be important. For some, particularly those in the early part of their careers, deciding on what they wanted out of a working life was problematic in the extreme. The dilemma of being able to choose seemed worse than having no choice at all. Whereas the path to completion of vocational training was quite clear, the direction thereafter seemed uncertain. Young doctors are confronted with an array of working opportunities including partnerships, assistantships, academic posts, associateships, salaried posts and retainer schemes. They want to know the advantages and disadvantages of full-time work, part-time work and job sharing. Mentoring offered them the chance to clarify their own priorities and make more in the way of plans than they perhaps had done up until that time.

In the course of the first meetings it became evident that some mentees had fairly low self-esteem. Instilling confidence and restoring self-esteem seems central to successful mentoring. By reaffirming a sense of worth mentors help mentees examine their own boundaries and take the risks necessary to move forward. Mentees may have been trying for some time to overcome an obstacle in their professional path without much success. The positive nature of the 'reflective' cycle enables mentees to place their past and current experiences in the context of their thoughts on the future. By bringing together the strands of their lives they can sometimes interpret events around them in a less damaging way. I could see that at times the mentees' distress led them to become isolated. They may become separated from their usual sources of support at work and even at home.[14] Mentoring can provide the encouragement necessary for doctors to rebuild their social and professional networks. Restoring their sense of worth is one of the key roles of mentoring. Confident doctors who value themselves can match aspirations to achievement and improve their life, rather than setting their sights too low.

Striving to be a good mentor

Mentoring is not always successful and being a mentor is not always a positive experience. Consistently being a good mentor sometimes seems an insurmountable task. As medical students and young doctors we are immersed in competition and ambition. Shedding these primordial mantles takes time and may not be complete. It is the recognition of that residual 'toxic' element in all of us that is perhaps of greatest importance on the path to becoming a good mentor.

A poor mentor can be too directive, opinionated, dogmatic, negative, a poor communicator, a poor listener, insensitive, disorganized and a poor time manager. I was aware of some of these failings during my mentoring. I was occasionally directive when I knew I should not have been. It was not always possible to be organized in the face of a mentee with complex and multiple agendas. I tried very hard to keep my own agendas out of the meetings but sometimes failed to do so. I sometimes offered advice or comment when silence would have immeasurably better, and sometimes stumbled into sensitive areas when clearly not invited.

I would sometimes fear the worst if a mentee was a few minutes late and would engage in merciless self-reproach. I quickly came to realize how emotionally exposed I was by mentoring. It challenged my self-confidence. In the very early days of the project I became conscious of my extreme inexperience as a mentor and worried about 'failing' in these particular relationships. Occasionally a relationship would come to an end or simply lapse into a dormant state without any obvious sign that it was going to do so. Feedback mechanisms were not always sensitive enough to pick up on why this might have happened and I was left guessing why things turned out the way they did. I was relieved to hear of similar experiences happening to other mentors but have learned a lot from some of the mistakes I thought I made in the beginning.

Support and accountability

The support framework for mentors in South Thames Region (West) has been central to the maintenance of a cohesive mentoring team. As a whole team mentors meet twice a year, and always finish with a team dinner. In addition we attend local support group meetings every 2–3 months and attend mentor development days on a termly basis.

The larger meeting looks mainly at our overall regional mentoring strategy. External speakers are invited to address the whole group on subjects ranging from reflective action planning to the healing powers of touch. Mentors from other regions sometimes attend these meetings, and then our comparison of experiences can prove illuminating, and has shown us several interpretations of mentoring. In my view these alternative models seem to resemble counselling or educational supervision more closely than they do mentoring. The possibility of linking mentoring to reaccreditation has been in the background of most discussions that have taken place during these particular days with most mentors strongly opposed to any such move.

Presenting our work at the last national mentoring conference brought me face to face with questions from delegates about whether or not mentoring should form part of a model of reaccreditation, how mentoring should be made accountable, how outcome should be measured and, very importantly, what funding arrangements should be adopted. When our project ended as a research study the Postgraduate Dean funded the scheme, reimbursing mentors £100 for their mentor sessions. In addition, both mentor and mentee were entitled to claim hours towards the Postgraduate Education Allowance (PGEA). From the postgraduate deans attending the conference came the clear message that whilst there was broad support for the concept of holistic mentoring they, in particular, require evidence of accountability as well as effectiveness before committing large amounts of public money to mentoring programmes on an ongoing basis.

The introduction of regional criteria for both mentors and mentees was undertaken through discussion between the mentor team and the Postgraduate Dean during a developmental meeting, in which the Postgraduate Dean spoke of the need to provide accountability, and suggested a regional agreement similar to that which exists for GP trainers and GP tutors. Nevertheless, when the criteria were introduced, it worried some mentors, and created tensions. It felt restrictive. The regional criteria specify the obligations of mentors in respect of training and mentoring practice as well providing guidelines for mentees. This was intended to make clear our commitment to the scheme, but was introduced at a time when some of us were feeling the strain of our existing commitment. The most controversial measure it seemed was the idea of a formal review at the end of four meetings, with a limit on the number of meetings that can occur annually per mentee. This was the inevitable result of funding limitations and, after discussion at local and regional group level, it became clear that there was greater flexibility in this area than the written criteria displayed, softening the blow of our new accountability. But it was still unacceptable to some, and three mentors left the team as a result. It is interesting to see that they are being replaced with mentees who have now, in their turn, become mentors and who will undertake a formal induction programme.

The local group meetings form the background of support for mentors. Our group of six/seven mentors meets regularly in the evening. At times, encouraged by the educational adviser, a mentor presents to other members of the group a mentoring encounter using a case study approach to reflective practice. This entails some preparation on the part of the presenter, who has to think carefully through their mentoring encounter, and give a reasonably detailed description of their interaction with their mentee. The intention is to share with each other how we go about conducting our session, what we learn from our actions, and gather input from colleagues which might inform and help us manage the mentor role effectively. At other times, we have a less structured discussion on the highlights and lowlights of being a mentor – for example, at a local support meeting recently a group of mentors set out the positive and negative aspects of being a mentor:

Positive	**Negative**
Feel good about doing it	Taking on problems
Improved professional treatment of doctors	Missing cues
Explored new areas	Unsatisfactory feelings
Increased understanding of practice problems	Going wrong
Greater insight into those we work with	Lack of feedback
Putting own problems into perspective	Too much emotional involvement
Meeting other mentors	Dependency culture
Exposure to new ideas	Restrictive criteria

We can then develop some ideas between us about how to address some of these aspects, and these meetings provide a useful and regular point to exchange information and learn from one another's experiences.

Reflections on experience

After over 2 years' mentoring I remain committed to its continuing development. I share the sentiment that there are 'personal dimensions of the mind and spirit' not addressed by our medical training.[15] My experience as a mentor to seven mentees has changed the way I look at myself and those whom I work with. The honesty of mentees and their clear expression of trust continues to intrigue me and underlines more than any other aspect of the process the acceptability of mentoring potentially to the whole profession.

The concept of a mentor as 'a dream facilitator' continues to fascinate me.[16] To bring alive the innermost ambition of an individual is tempting in the extreme. We all spend much of our lives entangled in intricate personal and professional webs and rarely have the opportunity to reflect on where we are now and where we wish to be in the years to come. Before a career can change, an individual needs to be able to voice the need for that change. Mentors, by setting aside their own agendas and through the use of the holistic model, provide a potential conduit for this self realization to take place. Mentoring is not only supportive and nurturing but also evoking of subconscious aspirations.

Being a mentor has enabled me, in a minor way, to give something back to a profession that has given me so much. Although in its infancy in medicine I am certain that mentors will become as much a part of everyone's lives as they have done in commerce and education. The cost in terms of training and protected time may be high, and intrinsic linkage with professional reaccreditation inevitable, but the potential for personal development is, in my view, enormous.

The second mentor's tale

Peter Harborow

As I first listened to Rosslynne Freeman's presentation on 'Mentoring for general practitioners', my enthusiasm was hooked into my being an active participant in the South West Thames mentoring programme. As I have been a trainer for several years, and have a diploma in counselling, the concept captured my imagination. I wanted to know more.

My own experience of medical education had varied from being humiliating in medical school to authoritarian, haphazard and lonely in hospital practice. When I arrived in general practice, I was fortunate to have partners who were interested enough to support me and moral enough not to exploit me. Taking annual study leave was considered imperative and ideas brought back were viewed favourably. I was actually surprised that they valued my opinion. This was refreshing.

Now, with increased pressures from the organizational aspects of general practice, patient demand, and long hours, it is all too easy to deny one's own needs and settle for the option of dealing with crises with blinkered fire-fighting. If not recognized it is a recipe for stress and burnout with possible disastrous consequences. Whilst money is of some importance, time spent developing supportive relationships, recognizing new opportunities, and planning for personal and professional development can ameliorate the condition. In the absence of a career structure in general practice, it is important for the individual to formulate his or her own strategies for self-evaluation and learning.

Modelling the mentor process

My role model in mentoring must have been my house-master at school. He spent individual time with each of the adolescent pupils, not teaching, but allowing the 'space' for them to explore and evaluate their own needs and to make plans and establish goals for the future. It was not until a long time afterwards that I realized the value of his interventions. I think this can apply also to the mentoring process.

Like mentoring programmes in other professions, the emphasis is on personal and professional development in a relationship of support and sometimes advocacy. It includes the strands of educational activity, all aspects of practice management and personal life management. These are inevitably intertwined and getting the balance right is essential. The mentor/mentee relationship is unique and provides a forum for exploration and decision making, where time out is taken for reflection.

The mentor/mentee relationship

Central to mentoring is the mentor/mentee relationship. As a mentor, I have valued each mentee. I have appreciated the special nature of each encounter and respect the position of trust in which the mentees have placed me. As a mentee myself, I have felt and received the unconditional positive regard imperative of such a relationship. The development of open, flexible, and genuine discourse with respectful challenge in an atmosphere of trust and protected time leads to finding a greater understanding of personal and professional aspects of life and enables the mentee to make changes, which will be beneficial. It is for the mentor to view the mentee's life 'as if' it were his/her own, without losing the 'as if' quality, to quote Carl Rogers.[17]

Setting the boundaries

Matching mentees with mentors has been successfully done via the project co-ordinator. It is important to start the relationship with no knowledge of each other. It eliminates bias and preconception and allows for an equal peer-level meeting. Having the practices close enough for ease of travelling, but far enough away for confidentiality, has worked very well. I have preferred to meet either in my home or that of the mentee.

The sessions have generally been for about one and a half hours. I think that is about the right length of time. To be professional, boundaries of confidentiality, timing and arrangement of meetings need to be observed. It differs very much from a chat or friendship, in as much as the mentor's own agenda is left behind and the session is strictly mentee centred. Meeting outside the session socially is not helpful as it alters the focus from the mentee to mentor. When, more recently, I decided to become a mentee within the scheme, as well as being a mentor, it meant that occasionally, I have met my mentor at the mentor developmental days, which always end socially, but this has not created a problem.

Getting started

Often the first session is exploratory. It is unusual for doctors to place themselves in the position of having an hour and a half, purely centred on their own issues. With this new experience the question of 'where do I begin?' often emerges. It is reassuring to know that there really is no right place to begin. Sometimes it is the first time that the mentee has had a chance just to 'off-load'. It is quite empowering just to do that. Where there is initial difficulty I have found the developmental cycle invaluable as a basis for getting started. It has the advantage of covering a great deal of ground very quickly in a structured manner. Being structured does not necessarily imply inflexibility. It enables the mentee to focus on personal and professional issues and to create a specific agenda with which he or she can work during the session rather than rambling on. At the end of each session the agenda can be revisited to see whether the items have been addressed and how the session went.

Mentoring is not counselling by another name. Although I have been involved in counselling for some years and consider that the use of counselling skills is fundamental to mentoring, I believe that the sessions should not become therapeutic. Nor should the sessions be just for teaching. However, during the interview every aspect of the mentee's life is up for consideration should he/she so wish. At times I have touched on both the therapeutic and the educational extremes in being able to offer genuine and useful support.

As a mentor, I do not set out to solve others' problems nor do I see it my place to offer advice as such. Sometimes it is reasonable to offer information, if I have it, and it is requested. In the first instance, being able to listen to an evolving story and to provide an atmosphere that contains it, just sort of keeps hold of it, is all that has been necessary. Usually, the agendas of my mentees have been of no surprise – they are quite often similar to mine. However, there are some important and individual differences. It is the mentee's issues that we are there to address. What I can do is to be there in an impartial and containing way with no personal bias and my own agenda on the shelf for that time. I may then be able to help them work out their own solutions, always remembering that any solutions are theirs, not mine.

One striking theme that emerges for me is that while many mentees cope with their practice in a very imaginative and apparently efficient way, there is still a strong sense of dissatisfaction. Delving deeper into the issues, there is adequate provision for dealing with emergent crises and reacting to patient and service demand, but this overshadows a real sense of the self and takes time away from setting and achieving personal and professional goals. In this sense, partnership problems, staffing relationships, and educational needs get overlooked until they themselves become crises. It is towards encouraging the mentee away from mere reacting to practice, which it cannot be denied is necessary at times, towards formulating proactive attitudes and plans which can be sustainable for the ensuing years of living. Reframing in that way and establishing a method of getting one's own needs met reduces that sense of dissatisfaction.

Building a trusting relationship

Rather like counselling, I believe that the mentor should demonstrate the basic qualities, as described by Carl Rogers, of unconditional positive regard or acceptance, empathy and genuineness. This is essential in helping the mentee express his/her agenda in a non-judgmental atmosphere. From my own experience as a mentee it is that fear of being thought silly or ignorant that holds me back from expressing my own concerns. Thus they may remain unaddressed. The stigma of seeking help for whatever reason as a doctor is often instilled in us in early medical school. It is the patients who have problems! Overcoming the fear of stigma may ease the first approach to a mentoring scheme. It takes time to build a trusting relationship and that trust of the mentor is essential for the success of mentoring. When the core conditions are met and trust established, a useful degree of respectful challenge is needed to help move on the mentee. Too little challenge and the mentee may remain 'stuck'. Too much and the mentee may feel vulnerable and attacked, the trust may be eroded and he/she may not want to continue. I find it important to check this out as we go along. Careful monitoring of response to probing open questions will discover no-go areas and these should be respected. If mentees have decided not to continue, I wonder if it is that I have been too challenging.

Setting the agenda

Using the developmental cycle model helps to delineate the broad range of issues that can be brought to the session by the mentee. I find this particularly useful when there is difficulty getting started. It does ensure that no area or topic is omitted and implies the broad nature of the mentoring process. This enables the mentee to work out his/her own agenda, which then forms the basis of the session or sessions. Generally issues fall into three categories: personal, professional, educational. Focusing down on a manageable agenda is important. Attempting to cover too much in one session results in nothing being achieved.

Structuring the work

As an adjunct to the developmental cycle, I have made much use of the Three Stage Model, described by Gerard Egan.[18] Briefly, he highlighted three stages:

1. Exploration of present scenario
2. Exploration of preferred scenario
3. Working out strategies for getting from 1 to 2.

These stages can be applied to any of the general areas and help to focus further. In stage one exploration, I have been entrusted with the wide richness of others' experience. It is a privilege to be there. This experience is often very positive and support seems to encourage further positive development. In elucidating negativity, it may be tempting to join in with an 'ain't it awful' and commiserate with the difficulties of medical practice. Focusing on negative aspects and working out strategies for improving them is more helpful.

Exploration of the present scenario can take some time and I find it important to devote some energy to getting a fuller picture of how the mentee thinks, feels and functions. Reflecting it back is a good way of helping the mentee get an understanding of her/his own process. Knowledge of how the mentee has arrived at the present situation may also shine light on the next stage: how to change it. Past successes, failures, role models and ideals all feature strongly in both helping the mentee to move forward and not to remain in the present situation.

Addressing the content

I cannot discuss content in any specific way, as I totally respect the concept of confidentiality. In general terms though, I have learned through both my sessions as a mentee and as a mentor, that the issues that confront us as doctors are similar. Often it is not a huge change that is necessary to resolve them, but a change in the way in which problems are viewed.

At the educational end of the spectrum of mentoring, uncovering and dealing with educational blocks is often more important than deciding and arranging which courses to go on. Partnership problems, staff difficulties, and patient demands could be helped by the mentees becoming aware of their own contribution to the difficult situations, and learning improved communication skills. It is then possible to evolve working more proactive strategies for how to achieve a balance between work, self, and home.

Addressing process

As Pallas Athene appeared to Odysseus and Telemachus in the guise of Mentor, there was a strong element of directive counselling. The aim of mentoring is to be non-directive and mentee centred. The concept of a mentor being 'older and wiser' should also be taken in perspective. The nature of the relationship is that it should be equal, between peers and that there should be no power differential. I try to avoid being paternalistic, although I think this is difficult for doctors. This could engender dependency or even worse symbiosis, where the mentor and mentee become interdependent. Transference and counter-transference, where both parties are playing out previous relationships, does not play a strong part in mentoring but it is useful to be aware of its possible presence. The daily round of doctoring encourages us to become rescuers and it is important to recognize this in the mentoring relationship. It lays the relationship open to becoming a game, like 'ain't it awful', 'why don't you . . . yes but . . .' in the sense of 'games people play' by Eric Berne.[19] Not entering the drama triangle allows for a more open relationship. It is also necessary in this context to leave one's own agenda on a back burner and not fall prey to over-identification. Although I know that in the longer run it is more empowering for mentees to work out their own solutions, at times I have sensed disappointment in some of my mentees that I am not offering a ready solution to their problems.

Setting goals

For mentoring to be effective it is necessary for the mentee to set some goals. In the early stages the goal may only be to decide what the goals are. To achieve a personal, professional or educational goal, it should be achievable and the result clear. If this goal is too large, it should be devolved into smaller bite-size chunks. During goal setting, it is necessary to address the demands that the individual places on him/herself. Those demands can be excessive. Sometimes it is those demands which drive his/her frenetic activity within working life which stop the consideration of and achievement of those goals. The mentor session enables the mentee to have space to view, set and achieve realistic goals. In this way, the knowledge of what may sabotage those goals can also be discovered. Often it is time taken up simply dealing with immediate practice problems. The mentor offers support and a chance to evaluate after putting the goals into action. I am really heartened by seeing mentees with whom I have worked making changes and achieving goals that they would not have imagined possible. It is difficult to see what I have done. It is the mentees who have done the work and made the changes. We only meet on a 2-monthly basis, but it I think it helps to bring into awareness innate resources of the individual.

Educational aspects

I was concerned that my preference towards counselling would bias the way in which I mentored; that I would concentrate too much on the psychological and therapeutic end of mentoring. On the contrary, while I have been wide open to that aspect I have very much enjoyed and been involved with working out individual educational plans with my mentees. This is rather like portfolio learning but then there are two people interested in it. I hope it is supportive.

I have used established methods of identifying patients' unmet needs (PUNS) and doctors' educational needs (DENS), both in my own education and in my mentees'. They do focus attention to the educational aspects of mentoring. Examining preferred ways of learning and being involved in someone else's ongoing process is exciting.

Finding support

If mentoring can be seen as a way of professional, personal, and educational supervision and support, so must the mentoring process itself be supported. Meeting in groups every 2 months has been really useful. It means not having to shoulder the whole responsibility of the process. It provides a forum for interchange of ideas about mentoring. Colleagues can point out issues that may have been missed and suggest other techniques that may be useful. I have received very useful feedback. This helped me to develop the way in which I mentor and to feel supported in this role.

I have also supplemented this by attending courses on mentoring. These courses widen my network, and cross-fertilization throughout this type of activity encourages my own further development of a personal style of professional mentoring. I have used my own knowledge of counselling and have gained assistance from my counselling supervisor where necessary. All of this stops isolation, which is one of the difficulties of general practice. I value any assistance to my development as a mentor, although the confidentiality of the mentoring session itself is always paramount.

Developing the model

The development of the model has been interesting. The developmental cycle has increased in its richness and complexity the more we have used it. Each member of the mentor team adds new perspectives. We have held developmental days and support days with outside speakers with interesting input into the project. The support group has also enhanced the model and made it more user-friendly. Each mentor's experience is valuable. I have also valued working with mentors from other regions. It widens my base of other issues, for instance gender and racial issues, and makes me appreciate other difficulties which mentors have experienced. I was surprised at the efforts to which some mentors went towards 'learning' in order to 'teach' the mentee. An important aspect of our meeting for me has been to form a network of support.

Training to be a mentor

Our training relies implicitly on the wide ranging skills that general practitioners have in being with and communicating with patients and colleagues. It is further extended by the understanding of the developmental cycle and the experiential practice of that model on training days. This is combined with the support network. My own interest in counselling and stress management has informed my mentoring. It has increased my active listening skills. However, I feel is not essential to have these extra qualifications. I think it is important to be able to recognize when these skills are necessary, perhaps where substance abuse, mental illness or stress likely to affect patient management may arise. Referral to a relevant agency would become appropriate. Mentoring is not an appropriate place for counselling or psychotherapy. Perhaps it would be useful to add to the training programmes some basic knowledge of stress and time management, and assertiveness techniques. I would value more knowledge and understanding of the educational process.

Record keeping and payment

I have maintained my own notes and keep them in a locked filing cabinet. I believe in the imperative of confidentiality. In the interests of accountability it is now necessary to send some communication to the team leader. This document is in the form of the mentor/mentee interview recording sheet. I fill this in at the end of each session and it contains only the information that both parties are happy to communicate to a third party. I feel that being paid is reasonable for the time and effort expended. If this scheme is as widely accepted and instituted as it may become, it could then become part of the educational/practice expenses through GMS. I am sure that mentoring should not be used as a reaccreditation method. It would alter the process from being mentee-led to policing. It could help while preparing for reaccreditation, in re-evaluating practice for the individual and getting over the hurdles, but confidentiality should be maintained.

A personal note

I have gained great personal benefit from being in the mentoring scheme. It has enabled me to build up my own network of support and have my own mentoring. It has enriched my own understanding of my profession and the people who work in it. Whilst helping others to change perspectives it also provides the opportunity to do the same for myself. It has assisted me to identify my own problem areas and, with the help of my mentor, consider aspects of practice that I would otherwise not have considered. At times it has been difficult to fit in all the activity that mentoring has involved. To do it properly does take time and commitment. I hope that mentoring schemes will continue and expand in the future. I think that they could form a firm foundation for personal and professional development for the individual, but on a larger scale it increases both motivation and expertise, which is very good overall for patient management, which is what we are in the business of providing. I think my experience over the last 3 years has been worthwhile and I hope that it has been worthwhile for my mentees.

These two accounts show something of the nature of becoming a mentor, and how the task was experienced. They are followed by four, briefer accounts from mentees, which give a flavour of being on the receiving end of the mentor's intervention. Although they are not named, all four of these mentees volunteered to write something of their experience, knowing that it was intended for publication.

In the first account, traces of the 'fortuitous relationship' are seen – the mentee is male, in his mid-thirties:

'The information about the mentor scheme fell on my desk when I had just gone through a partnership split, and had been ill prior to that. I was quite low, and I think the timing was right for me. I wanted someone independent with whom I could discuss my work, the workload and various projects, but also my time off. It's not easy to get back into the swing of things when you have been off ill.

What did we talk about? Mostly getting the balance between work – the working week and personal time – right. We talked about my taking on various new projects, but this led to discussing how I could become more selective, and keep a better balance, so that I had time to myself. Mentoring showed me that I needed to learn to say "no" – and not to feel guilty about it.

Meeting at each other's surgeries was a good idea, and we worked through a list of things, professional and personal, although I did not feel comfortable enough with my mentor to discuss things of a really personal nature, like family issues. Getting feedback on things was a very positive and helpful aspect of mentoring.

What qualities do mentors need? I think they should be non-judgmental – that's very important in the relationship; also not to have fixed ideas – they need to be flexible. They should know where to draw the line, and not probe too deeply, which can be embarrassing. Also they need to remain independent, and not become involved. Mentors should also be able to cover all sorts of issues, professional and personal if necessary. Family medicine is changing rapidly, and different models will become the "norm" – mentors need to be able to accept all the different ways of working, according to the needs of their mentee, male or female – this flexibility of thought is essential.'

For another male mentee, similar in age, this question of career patterns and finding ways of developing a career was the factor which prompted him to take up the offer of a mentor:

'There is such a lack of support for career development in general practice. I could see no good forum for personal development type issues and, for me, mentoring provided this focus.

But that was not all that I discussed with my mentor, although I suppose other issues such as partnership problems and team working were related to my main theme of personal and career development. I also talked about balancing work and family life and, through these discussions, I gained an objective and (hopefully) a wise alternative view on a number of current life and work problems. I found what was very helpful in the mentoring meeting was the reflective-type counselling, and advice on other options available to me. A good empathic mentor was invaluable to me at that time.

I think it is vitally important that mentors are able to have empathy, objectivity, and are able to challenge assumptions in a non-patronizing way. I also think experience in general practice is necessary, to engender respect. For me, mentoring was a valuable part of career support in the context of lifelong learning, and personal development. I think *every* GP, and probably every doctor, should have a mentor.'

In this account the mentee had, it seemed, come to his mentor with a clear idea of the career development issues that were on his agenda. But occasionally, mentees come with less certain ideas and then find that events overtake them, and become the focus of their working agenda. When this happens, the relationship is indeed fortuitous; it exists as a valid place to take a developing crisis and this illustration, provided by a young female doctor who worked with a female mentor, offers a vivid glimpse of how that might happen:

'When I joined the mentoring scheme I had no really clear idea of what I wanted to use my mentor for beyond the usual stuff of practice politics – it seemed like a good idea, and there is certainly not enough support for GPs once they have left training. In the first couple of meetings we were getting to know each other, but over time many changes occurred in my practice which were very stressful and difficult. On top of all of that, I had an accident, and was quite badly injured. I remember very clearly one night, quite late, when I was really at rock bottom – I could see no way out, beyond leaving general practice for good. The phone rang and it was my mentor – she told me she had been doing the ironing and suddenly felt quite strongly that I was in trouble – I couldn't believe it, the timing was incredible, it was magic! After that call, we met quite quickly, and once I off-loaded the immediate awfulness, we met 2-monthly, and worked through an agenda which included communication skills, managing confrontations with difficult partners, and my future career.

Mentoring began to put the buzz back into general practice. My mentor gave me alternative views, and suggested other options which I had not thought about.

I started to keep a learning diary. Gradually I have restructured my future, I am doing a higher degree, and have found a different pattern of clinical work. I am no longer in a crisis, and do not feel I need to see my mentor that frequently. The trouble is when you are overwhelmed, you can't imagine that you have time to see a mentor, yet someone who feels that probably needs one more than most. The actual time input is only a couple of hours a month.

I think I was extremely lucky with my mentor; she had quite special insight. Not all mentors need it in such a high degree, but I think mentors do need to put the interests of their mentee first, and care enough about their future to pay attention to them. Another important thing is that my mentor comes from outside my practice environment, and so can take a dis-passionate look at my viewpoint. A second head can often come up with an alternative solution, from a different angle. I get the benefit of experience that someone else has learnt the hard way!

I have had tremendous educational benefit in the broadest sense of the word. An indirect result of mentoring has been to identify my sources of stress, and sort some of them out, thus releasing "mind-space" to take on new challenges, like my MSc. Mentoring identified my strengths and weak-nesses, clarified my thinking, and helped me plan some goals. Mentoring is not a threatening experience, but it is certainly a challenging one. However, for someone who was on the verge of leaving general practice, I now think my professional life is fantastic!

I hope that this is only the start of mentoring – a pebble dropped into a pool from which ripples will spread outwards. Those of us who have benefited may in time become mentors ourselves. There is a wealth of experience in our profession in caring for others it is about time we started to look after each other.'

It seemed that the availability of a mentor when the storm broke was an important aspect of this mentee's experience. Once the catharsis of crisis was over, she could settle into planning a different future. Yet, more often, mentees come because they simply want someone to talk to, as our fourth mentee, the only woman in an otherwise all-male partnership recounts:

'I took up mentoring because I have always felt that we GPs need to "unload" our feelings to someone who understands our unique problems. The only way this can be achieved is for GPs to talk to each other, in a similar way to counsellors, who co-counsel each other.

I have discussed all sorts of things with my mentor, from childcare to locality commissioning. The most useful discussions have been in areas involving partnership disputes, and problems with patients. We have discussed time management within surgeries, how to handle difficult patients, and had some fascinating discussions on the different problems of male and female doctors!

My mentor has always been useful – I understand now why people go to their GPs! It has been wonderful to talk to someone who listens so well, and is completely non-judgmental. He has years of experience, and has made the same mistakes, so can offer wise advice, as well as point me in the right direction when he can't provide the answers I want.

Obviously, my mentor is not perfect, and often problems have no answer, but I have found discussing these problems to be helpful, just to confirm that I am doing my best in trying to solve them.

I think mentors need particular qualities – they need to be good listeners, and have an open mind. I have found it helpful that he has plenty of experience, is unafraid to give me personal advice and to draw, at times, on his own personal experience. Not being judgmental or easily shocked is important, as is the ability to give that is open to negotiation. These are all the qualities of a good GP!

I hope mentoring goes from strength to strength. Mentors themselves need their own guidance, help and support. I would love to see all new GPs being offered mentoring, as well as it being more widely available to older GPs. The fact that mentors have no prior knowledge of the mentee is important, but travelling can be difficult and time consuming. Mentoring takes time ironically, at the times when I've been most stressed and in need of my mentor I have least time to see him!'

In the beginning of the mentor's tale, taking on the role of a mentor, and beginning mentoring relationships with their peers was likened to Pandora's story, as she released from the forbidden jar every ill, trouble and sin into the world of general practice. It is timely to recount the end of her story when, as she moped around the house in disgrace from her meddling, she miserably took another look into the empty jar. As she did, a beautiful winged creature, who had been trapped under the lid, fluttered out. Pandora immediately felt a lightening of mood, an uplifting of her spirits. Without knowing it she had left hope trapped in the jar, and had now released it to fly into the world and become humanity's solace against despair.

At this stage in our story it seems that, like Pandora, things are not as bad as was feared. The main protagonists – the mentors and their mentees – having mastered their initial anxieties and opened the jar, find hope lying trapped underneath various troubles. They release it to overcome many obstacles in their path, and are now proceeding steadily on their way. But, of course, it is the prerogative of story tellers to believe utterly in the tale they are telling and, in so doing, invite the listeners to collude in their perception of events. The following chapter should restore the balance, and like a good mentor, offer at times an alternative view of the mentoring journey.

References

1 Longhurst M. 1988 Self-awareness – the neglected insight. *Canadian Medical Association Journal,* **139**, 121–4
2 Merriam S. 1983 Mentors and proteges – a critical review of the literature. *Adult Education Quarterly,* **33**(3), 161–73
3 Hagerty B. 1986 A second look at mentors. *Nursing Outlook,* **34**(1) 16–24
4 Beecham L. 1997 BMA calls for 10% pay increase for doctors. *British Journal of Medicine,* **315**, 698
5 Cooper C.L. and Sutherland V.J. 1992 Job stress, job satisfaction, and mental health among general practitioners before and after the introduction of the new contract. *British Medical Journal,* **304**, 154–8
6 Freeman R. 1995 Mentoring in general practice. *Education for General Practice,* **7**, 112–7
7 Perkoff G.T. 1992 To be a mentor. *Family Medicine,* **24**, 584–5
8 Levinson D. *et al.* 1978 *The Seasons of a Man's Life.* Knopf, New York
9 Ibid
10 Klug B.J. and Salzman S.A. 1991 Formal induction vs. informal mentoring – comparative effects and outcomes. *Teaching and Teacher Education,* **7**, 241–51
11 Ibid 1995
12 Ibid
13 Francis D. 1994 *Managing Your Own Career.* Harper Collins, London
14 Chambers R. 1993 Avoiding burnout in general practice. *British Journal of General Practice,* **43**, 442–3
15 Thomasma D.C. 1982 A cognitive approach to the humanities in primary care. *Family Medicine,* **14**(4), 18–20
16 Ibid
17 Rogers C. 1990 *On Becoming A Person,* 2nd edn. Constable, London
18 Egan G. 1990 *The Skilled Helper,* 5th edn. Brookes/Cole, Pacific Grove CA
19 Berne E. 1964 *Games People Play.* Penguin

———7———

Evaluating the mentor scheme

'Where is the life we have lost in living?
Where is the wisdom we have lost in knowledge?
Where is the knowledge we have lost in information?'

(T.S. Eliot[1])

> Part 1 of this chapter opens with a summary of the action-research framework of the mentor scheme, and gives reasons why this methodology was selected as being appropriate to the activity of mentoring. This is followed by a short account of the outcomes of the internal evaluation, carried out by the scheme leader. However, the main emphasis in the chapter comes in part two, and is provided by independent researchers who were commissioned to undertake an external evaluation of the work of the second mentor team, who tell how they went about their task, and offer a further example of a model of evaluation for use in mentoring.

Part 1: False divisions in research methodology

Earlier in this story reference was made of the false divide between thinking and feeling, so powerfully introduced in medical training. If, when designing a model of holistic mentoring an anticipated outcome could have been identified, it would be encapsulated in the hope that mentoring could reconcile this false divide, by restoring the authenticity of feelings and returning practitioners to a more holistic view of their personal and professional selves.

In keeping with this, the evaluation methodology through which information was gathered on the impact of mentoring in professional life needed to be placed within a research framework which in itself created no false divide between thinking and feeling, and in its underpinning philosophy, held in equal value knowledge gained of both the personal and the professional self. It needed to be a framework which supported our efforts to gain knowledge and understanding from the active *practice* of the mentoring role, and the *process* of the mentoring relationship itself.

This was a central feature in determining the various ways in which the data were gathered and interpreted, all of which were based in the daily routines of delivering the mentor scheme to general practitioners. The mentor support groups and their developmental days, in addition to their supportive, educational focus acted as a focus group,[2] where interaction between the mentors encouraged them to develop and explore their own questions about mentoring and develop a framework for understanding. The themes emerging from the mentor groups were noted by the scheme leader, and later developed through individual semi-structured and depth interviews with randomly selected mentors. To maintain confidentiality, data from mentees was gathered anonymously, via the administrative structures of the scheme, using the 6-monthly feedback forms which asked about their experience of being mentored, and if they could identify outcomes of the intervention. Themes collated from these 6-monthly reviews were later followed up by focus groups with those mentees who agreed to attend. In this way, the consistent themes emerging from mentors were placed alongside consistent themes emerging from the mentees, providing a means of cross-checking the experience of both parties.

These methods supported the concept of grounded theory,[3] where data are not tested against any predetermined statement of theories, but rather allows for theory to be developed from observation and practice, and this same emphasis on practice-led theory is at the heart of action-research frameworks, defined by Elliott:[4]

'Action research might be defined as the study of a social situation with a view to improving the quality of action within it. It aims to feed practical judgement in concrete situations, and the validity of the "theories" or hypotheses it generates depends not so much on "scientific" tests of truth, as on their usefulness in helping people to act more intelligently and skilfully. In action research theories are not validated independently and then applied to practice – they are validated through practice' [my emphasis] (p. 69).

The action research perspective was born in 1960, arising from a sense of professional disenchantment in education not dissimilar to that which heralds the birth of mentoring in general practice today. The differentiation of educational provision between grammar and secondary schools prompted a critical response from secondary school teachers, frustrated by the irrelevant and inappropriate curricula which they were expected by the universities to deliver to their already-alienated pupils. It began as a professional reaction against the divide between theory and practice, voiced by teachers who had imposed upon them a syllabus irrelevant and inappropriate to need, and unworkable in practice. Their response will find echoes amongst those academics in medicine determined to wrest the undergraduate curriculum from its predominantly hospital context and provide for more relevant learning in the community, and can be understood by GPs antipathetic towards imposed protocols and guidelines handed down from above by those who stand apart from the reality of practice, particularly when, as with education in the 1960s, actions take place against a backdrop of imposed change.

Creative secondary school teachers constructed their response to an irrelevant syllabus through forming support groups. In these they strove to openly share those aspects of their personal practice which set about reinterpreting the set syllabus, and offered instead meaningful and relevant learning to their pupils. Some teachers worked across the boundaries of subjects as a teaching team, under models of leadership from their head teachers who supported change without coercion. Groups developed into supportive networks of practitioners committed to transforming an educational culture, through making explicit not only their practice but the beliefs and values that underpinned it.

Their work defined the fundamental attributes of action research, discernible in the unfolding description of mentors at work contained in previous chapters. In action research, 'theories' of teaching and learning are derived from attempts to bring about a change in a particular set of circumstances. They are not so much applications of theories learned from professional training, but attempts to make explicit theories derived from practice. The production and utilization of knowledge is subordinate to, and conditioned by, the fundamental aim of improving practice.

Improving practice involves jointly considering the quality of both process and outcomes – Schon's reflective practice. This aspect is seen in the model of the mentor support groups, where reflection on experience was followed by mentors making explicit their theories of practice, opportunistic teaching and discussion about 'academic' theories which might, or might not, offer differing perspectives.

A further attribute of action research is that it is conducted by practitioners, researching into areas of their own professional practice. This makes the role of practitioner and researcher inseparable. As Dadds[5] puts it:

'. . . to be a (practitioner) action researcher is to bring the existing self as a practitioner into the research process. And with it comes all the attendant wisdom, knowledge, beliefs, values, attitudes, prejudices, loves and hates of the personal and professional self. In practice . . . the practitioner lives inside the being of the researcher. The researcher lives inside the being of the practitioner . . . each informing, each shaping the other' (p. 229).

For Kemmis,[6] it is this first person focus that demarcates 'insider' action research from the traditional 'outsider' research, in which the research agenda is set and conducted by outsiders who have no direct involvement, or indeed particular interest in, the aspect being researched. This introduces one of the many aspects of action research likely to provoke a clash of professional cultures. Although there is a welcome shift in medicine towards acknowledging the complementary role of qualitative research,[7] with increasing acceptance that its interpretative, naturalistic approach to studying a phenomenon in its natural setting is appropriate for many topics, for many doctors 'validity' still lies in a rigorous, yet distant and objective quest for a 'right' answer arrived at through standardized tests of measurement.

Throughout this book my own personal experiences as a project leader and 'first person' researcher have been offered in an attempt to make my own practice explicit, and thereby accessible to others. It was done so knowing that some readers would find the infiltration of my personality into the work of the scheme uncomfortable, and lead them to question the validity of the evaluation findings.

If this aspect smacks of heresy, there's more to come. Action research not only challenges the sacred tenets of the researcher being an impartial actor who 'does' research 'on' others, but turns it on its head. Rather than see the involvement of the practitioner–researcher as a contaminating factor which thereby renders the research and its outcomes invalid, the personal involvement of the researcher is seen as a benefit, an illuminating force which, through the process of the practitioner making public their theories of enquiry, makes the outcomes *more* valid.

But the concept of the practitioner–researcher being one and the same is perhaps more easily tolerated when laid alongside the further distinction of action research, which lies in the commitment to action. Here the two professional cultures are united, as the objective of much qualitative research in medicine is to close the gap between the discovery of the 'right' answer, and actually putting it into practice, research which explores reasons as to why so much medical research fails to be implemented.

In this context, two research cultures are united by the dilemma of divisions – between theory and practice, the researcher and the researched, the researcher and their self. It might then be less than heretical to consider first-person research. When the main objective of the research is to bring about change or improvement in an area of professional practice, who better to drive the active pragmatic process which proposes and formulates an intervention, and then systematically monitors its application, than a practitioner? When the practitioner has ownership of the research agenda in this way, research and usage are not seen as separate entities, but as part of an integrated whole, a commitment to practical as well as conceptual views of new knowledge.

This integration of research and usage in action research calls forth the courage of practitioners to engage in a continuing process of reflection, not solely as a means of improving practice, but as a means of constantly reassessing the values on which that practice was based, and on which the outcome of the intervention is judged. Realizable values are context bound, and are ultimately a personal judgement.

In the first 18 months of the South Thames (West) mentor scheme, the 6-monthly review forms of the first intake of mentees (27 in all) were thematically analysed, and yielded some evidence of the value that they placed on the mentoring intervention,[8] and how these had become realizable in practice. Themes relating to the value of the mentor included:

The neutral, independent, objective status of the mentor
Availability of their support
The ongoing, continuing nature of the relationship
The mentor's ability to be both supportive and challenging
The professional structure of the relationship
Interpersonal skills of the mentor
The opportunity to talk freely and openly, without judgement.

The value of the mentoring intervention appeared realizable firstly in the mentees' changed view of themselves, and increased self confidence, which for the majority was an unexpected outcome, although this appeared to get worse before it got better. Mentees told how mentoring made them more aware of their own needs, which in turn brought a realization of the extent of their isolation and unhappiness, and the lack of ready, sustainable peer support. But this gave way to the realization that others in their profession felt as they did; they were not 'different' from their peers. This heralded the arrival of the 'feel good factor', which embraced statements about 'every doctor should have a mentor'. The changed view of self was then used to realize changes in practice. Through the process of the mentoring relationship, with its shared reflection on the various aspects of professional life, the mentees' energy and enthusiasm for general practice, obscured by time and events, was re-asserted. The realizable value of mentoring was then used to change and develop practice, instigating alternative ways of being. The mentor's continuing presence in the mentee's life served to assist the implementation of new practices, and then monitor and support the outcomes of change. This consistency appeared as another realizable value, described by one mentee in these words:

'mentoring made me realize that my career is NOW – not somewhere in the future'.

This same quality and continuous nature of the mentor's personal support resulted in strategies being defined to enhance coping mechanisms for the stress resulting from overload. The mentors' overt valuing of their mentees gave to many permission to value themselves:

'through my mentoring I came to recognize that I am a human being first and a general practitioner second'.

From this came the further usable value of empowerment. They took back control of their professional lives, and in so doing discovered their individual power which could be used to the good of the organization:

'instead of waiting impatiently for my partners to change, I saw that I could be the one to initiate change . . . so I did . . . and it worked.'

However, values are ultimately personal judgements, making it difficult to assess the value of change in personal attitudes and beliefs. Individually, I believed those mentees who said that mentoring changed their attitudes, and particularly their response to others, as it would naturally follow from a supportive relationship which has promoted insight and understanding. But, as the previous chapter on reflective practice shows, the very act of reflection transforms values, so that they constitute ever receding standards, tantalizingly out of reach. Personally, I consider that a doctor empowered to become a change-agent in their group practice is a 'good' outcome of mentoring, but this value might not be shared by partners who find that a previously docile colleague now actively demands change.

In one focus group, whilst the discussion set out to confirm the outcome themes shown in the review forms, further reflection on these made their value contentious. As the discussion developed, a member of the group described their mentoring experience, in which the mentor was described as 'brilliant – just what was needed' and was full of praise for the skills of a mentor who had been so accurately insightful, challenging, yet warm and supportive. But as the mentoring progressed, this mentee quite quickly realized that feelings of frustration over being a 'misfit' arose not from being in the wrong group practice, as had been surmised, but from being in the wrong job. This having been clarified, the mentee was in the process of leaving general practice to read art history. Was that a good outcome?, I asked the group. Did it foster the implicit values underpinning mentoring, which infer that promoting the wellbeing of practitioners ensures that they stick around and continue to deliver quality patient care?

This integration of research and usage further conveys an archetype of a research framework in which there are no false divisions, but an integration – of self into the researcher, the practitioner into the research, and the practice into the theory. It is a model admirably supported from inside the profession by Howie,[9] who addresses the credibility gap in general practice research, calling for better theory, more feeling, and less strategy. But the small size and limited budgets of mentor schemes and, in this research project, the emphasis on an integrated evaluation, defy the development of strategies which might enhance the credibility of this type of applied qualitative research.

Nevertheless, the rigorous work of the two mentor teams using the holistic model of mentoring continued to attract attention. The second mentor team, being differently positioned, had access to other funding, and by this means came a commission for an independent, external evaluation of their work. Whilst accepting the small-scale nature of this study, the appointed independent researchers brought with them a recognition of the potential growth of mentoring in medicine, a perspective which influenced the design of their evaluation to render it replicable. Writing from the position of independent researchers, they share here the design and outcome of their evaluation.

Part 2: Evaluating mentoring – an outside perception

Maria Ruegger
Elizabeth Sullivan

Introduction

In this second part of the chapter we describe our evaluation of a small mentoring project. It is our hope that in doing so, others who are undertaking a similar task will find this account of our experience informative. We will describe the way in which we approached the task, how we identified and chose the methods we used, and discuss the theoretical basis underpinning our methodology. In order to give the reader a flavour of both the process and the outcome of the evaluation, we describe some of the detail of our findings, discuss the conclusions we drew, and reflect on the limitations of a small scale study. Finally we offer some suggestions for further inquiry which became apparent to us as a result of our evaluation.

Deciding on a methodology for evaluation

Any evaluation must begin with the question, 'what precisely is to be evaluated?'[10] The methods chosen to conduct the evaluation will be dependent on the answer to this question. This question itself should be broken down into meaningful parts. Before we began to work on the evaluation discussed in this chapter, we sought answers to the following questions:

- For whom is the evaluation being undertaken, and for what purpose?
- Who or what is being evaluated?
- What is the environment in which the 'who' or 'what' are located?

FOR WHOM WAS OUR EVALUATION UNDERTAKEN AND FOR WHAT PURPOSE?

We found that our evaluation could be seen to meet the needs and interest of three groups. Firstly, the budget holding authority required information about the usefulness of the mentoring scheme. Secondly, the organizers of the mentoring scheme required information and feedback related to the many practical, methodological and theoretical issues of setting up and running the project. Thirdly, those participating in the mentoring scheme as mentors and mentees were interested in understanding the scheme in its entirety, and in contributing to its development.

The purposes of the evaluation became apparent once the three interested groups were identified. The budget holders needed information to enable them to make future funding decisions. It was important, therefore, that they chose independent evaluators whose impartiality to the material collected ensured an accurate reflection of the usefulness of the initial scheme. The organizers needed information to enable them to check how far the scheme was achieving what they intended it to. It was important here that the evaluators were aware of the organizers' intentions and their methods, so that the evaluation could elicit relevant information. The participants, whose collective views as reflected in the evaluation report might influence the future of the scheme, wanted to know the results of their contribution to the evaluation.

WHO OR WHAT IS BEING EVALUATED?

In this case 'who' refers to the mentors, whose performance in the role was evaluated by their mentees and, by implication, the project leader and organizers who prepared them for their new role. It also refers to the number of participants in the evaluation, which was very small in this case. The 'what' refers to the mentoring scheme for mentoring in general practice as a whole, and this was commented on by both mentors and mentees.

WHAT IS THE ENVIRONMENT IN WHICH THE 'WHO' OR 'WHAT' ARE LOCATED?

An evaluation should be alive to the environment in which a scheme such as this is operating. There was a large amount of cultural specificity (as opposed to diversity) in this group, across four dimensions: professional roles (all participants in the evaluation were GPs); organizational setting (all from the same health authority); geographical location (all from the same small, deprived city area); and ethnicity of participants (predominantly Asian). This knowledge shaped some of the questions asked, as will be seen later.

Armed with the information about what precisely was to be evaluated, we considered the methods best suited to the task. Such a small population of participants does not lend itself to quantitative methods of inquiry.

Rather, the evaluation of this scheme, which was developed using methods drawn from a qualitative approach, demanded a methodology which could capture emergent themes. The action research methods, referred to in this first part of this chapter, had been employed in the larger, South Thames (West) project to develop and support the implementation of mentoring, and these are located in a qualitative social research tradition.[11] The mentor team leader had used the mentor support groups as focus groups, and carried out some opportunistic, unstructured interviews with mentors to generate issues and themes from which the scheme evolved and developed. These focus groups provided the opportunity for mentors to 'observe' and 'describe' their actions, relationships, thoughts and feelings, and the resulting issues and themes were the basis of some of the questions used in the evaluation interview. Thematic analysis of participants' responses in the evaluation revealed much of the rich and complex nature of the mentoring experience, and allowed us to explore similarities and differences in their perceptions.

The evaluation

Our commission was to undertake a small scale study involving all GP mentees participating in a pilot mentoring scheme. Our task was to conduct an independent evaluation of the impact of mentoring on the professional development of GPs. Mentors had been available to GPs in their area for approximately 12 months, and twenty doctors had accessed this service by the time we began our evaluation. We also interviewed six of the twelve mentors participating in the scheme. The focus for this aspect of our study was the mentors' experience of mentoring, and the structure within which mentoring was arranged and supported. From a list of participating mentors we chose six at random.

The mentor scheme operated in a predominantly white, working class area, which is considered to be socially and economically deprived, with high levels of unemployment, poverty and family breakdown being common features. Consequently it is an area designated for special funding to support and promote general practice, together with a range of complementary educational activities. It was through this that funding was made available for the establishment of a mentoring scheme, and its evaluation.

All twenty of the GPs who had used the mentoring scheme agreed to participate in the evaluation. This is likely to have been influenced, in part, by the fact that funding was available to cover the costs of participants' professional time. GPs were able to claim amounts equal to that which they would need to arrange for locum cover in respect of the time they spent with their mentors/mentees; these same rates were available to cover time spent with the project evaluators. Another factor, which we believe is likely to have influenced the response rate, concerns the measures taken to give assurances to participants about the purpose of the evaluation, and the use to which the information they gave us would be put. In particular we were aware that those GPs who had used mentoring to discuss personal matters might be reluctant to be interviewed. We wrote to all GP mentees in advance to explain our involvement, what we expected of them and the measures being taken to ensure confidentiality. The letter stressed that the report had two purposes: firstly to provide information to the funding body, which might have implications for the allocation of future resources, and secondly to provide feedback to the scheme developers and organizers to influence the development of the scheme. We made it clear that the personal content of mentoring sessions was not being evaluated, and that the raw material would not be made available to the mentor scheme leader, to the Education Director who directed and commissioned her work, or to any other GP, or to any other person. We assured potential subjects that in our final report of the evaluation findings it would be impossible to distinguish individual responses.

Methods of evaluation

We devised two sets of interview questions, one for mentees and another for mentors. Questions were designed to facilitate comparisons between mentors' and mentees' responses. Both were administered during personal interviews which were recorded on tape. However, where GPs objected to the tape recording their answers were written down in detail, and checked with the interviewee for accuracy. We interviewed GPs in their surgeries, taking on average 45 minutes. The gender breakdown of the participants was as follows: four of the mentees were female, 17 male. Mentors comprised five male and one female.

The interview questions sought to obtain information on three distinct areas:

- Experience of being mentored or being a mentor
- Outcome of mentoring
- Structure within which mentoring was arranged and supported.

The questions aimed to produce qualitative information by facilitating mentors' and mentees' exploration of issues important to themselves. As independent evaluators we took into account the possibility of researcher bias, so we put in place systems to minimize the impact on both data collection and evaluation.[12] A pre-agreed series of prompts was associated with each question to guide subject responses. The taped interviews were exchanged by the evaluators for cross checking of analysis to ensure as far as possible a standard approach.

Process and outcomes of evaluation

MENTEES' EVALUATION

The first part of the interview was about the experience of being mentored. We asked recipients questions about how they had used the mentoring service, such as how often they had met with their mentors, for how long, and whether these variables influenced their satisfaction with the scheme. Their meetings lasted between 90 minutes and 2 hours, and the majority felt that meetings at bi-monthly intervals were about right. Satisfaction rates were only in part to do with regular use of the scheme, as some GPs felt that they had achieved their own personal objectives following just one session.

From a list of fifteen, mentees were invited to choose five characteristics which most closely reflected their view of their mentor. They were then asked to grade their mentor on those five characteristics using a given scale. The characteristics most admired by mentees were those of good listener, supportive colleague, trustworthiness and the ability to convey respect for others' opinions. The responses showed that there was a significant amount of agreement between mentees in relation to the characteristics they chose, and the scores show that there was a high level of satisfaction with mentors overall. Responses to a later question, which required mentees to draw a pen picture of an ideal mentor, revealed a close match with the characteristics they had earlier identified, and valued, in their own mentors.

We considered that gender and ethnicity might possibly be variables which could affect satisfaction rates. Initially we did not find these to be significant as the majority of mentees suggested that professional knowledge and experience were much more relevant. Where an opinion was expressed, in response to interviewer prompts, culture was held to be more important than gender on the basis that shared background and experience facilitates understanding and communication, and that mentors from a similar cultural background would have struggled with many of the same problems. Responses to this question did not appear to be affected by the gender or culture of the mentee.

A more important concern for mentees was the issue of confidentiality. Only four mentees said that they did not have concerns about this prior to joining the scheme. Worries were largely about the degree of confidentiality mentees felt they could expect. Generally however, it was felt that early concerns had been allayed. Most mentees reported that their mentor had raised the issue of confidentiality at the first meeting. This, together with several other factors, seemed sufficient to overcome early anxieties. Amongst these factors were that mentors were doctors, for whom confidentiality is second nature, and in many cases mentees had prior personal knowledge of, and respect for, their mentor. However, the comparatively small size of the geographical area made for close proximity in terms of the professional community from which mentees and mentors were drawn, and was a factor which seemed in some cases to have had a negative impact on the process of establishing a safe relationship with the mentor.

We wanted to know for what matters GPs saw mentoring as a potential solution. Popular areas for discussion with mentors included stress, stress related health problems, personal relationships and professional relationships, all of which featured prominently, followed by training needs and business matters.

The second phase of the interview dealt with the outcome of mentoring. All respondents identified a measure of positive outcome, although the extent varied. We found that a large number of minor changes in different areas could be perceived by mentees as amounting to a significant overall change, or that change was seen as occurring gradually through the process of being exposed to new ideas. All participants valued the opportunity for discussion, and this applied even when mentees were unable to identify changes resulting from mentoring.

When asked whether their valued outcomes could have been achieved without the services of a mentor, the majority felt that they could not. Similarly when asked whether they could suggest an alternative to the mentoring service which would have better meet their needs, mentees said that they could not. Sixteen of the respondents said they would unreservedly recommend mentoring to colleagues on the basis of their own experience, and the remaining five said that they would in some circumstances, and particularly to single-handed practitioners. When asked what they valued least about their mentoring experience some mentees commented that teaching was not helpful as there were other, better ways of meeting this need. Several commented that finding time was difficult, whilst others suggested that having to request mentoring, rather than it being part of everyone's career development, was an undesirable feature of the scheme.

We wanted to know mentees' views on how mentoring could best be used. There was strong support for mentoring to be available to all GPs and that it should be part of the career structure. The majority of mentees told us that, with the benefit of hindsight, they would not now hesitate to join the mentoring scheme.

The final part of the interview dealt with the structure within which mentoring is arranged and supported. All mentees wished to contribute suggestions for the development of the mentoring service. The main themes arising from their suggestions were:

- Mentoring should become part of a national framework of support for career development
- Mentoring, in the form of peer support by professional equals, should be introduced
- There was nothing to prevent GPs being mentors and mentees simultaneously
- Feedback from participants should inform the development of the service
- Training in counselling type skills for mentors should be provided
- A system for the selection of mentors following training should be devised.

There was almost unanimous support for the mentoring scheme to be extended, improved and made accessible to all.

The format of a questionnaire used to elicit the mentees' response to the impact of mentoring, which was part of our evaluation methodology, is included in the Appendices.

MENTORS' EVALUATION

The six mentors we interviewed had been offering a service in their area for between 12 and 18 months. They received three workshop based training sessions prior to taking on their first mentees. Subsequently they have attended six weekly support groups, supplemented at 3-monthly intervals by meetings of the entire group, facilitated by their project leader.

At times they had joined up with mentors from the South Thames (West) Region.

All six mentors talked about the dual benefit of helping their colleagues at the same time as helping themselves. All made some comment about the importance of the listening, helping and supporting aspects of mentoring, linking this with the idea of dedicating time to the process. There was a clear belief that the modern environment in which GPs operate causes many difficulties which were not dealt with in other ways. In a similar vein, some commented on the special culture of the general practitioner, which doesn't encourage individuals to seek help. Mentors appeared to make the assumption that the mentor scheme would enable GPs to overcome this reluctance to seek help and support.

Mentors told us that they found the training workshops and support groups useful for basic knowledge, professional development and the opportunity to practise skills. The workshops facilitated members' investment in, and sense of ownership of, the project. Several mentors likened the workshops and small groups to a form of mentoring for mentors, and thus it would seem that training workshops served a number of important functions. All six mentors thought that mentoring was enjoyable, and also worth the time and effort they put into it. Most of them were involved with between two and four mentees and this, in addition to the workshops and group meetings attended by all the mentors, represented a large commitment of time. It is unclear why the GPs who choose to be mentors appeared to have more time and less stress than those GPs who became mentees. All the mentors described the role as important in relation to their other professional commitments, and the reasons given were in terms of its perceived efficacy in stress reduction, and its inherent role satisfaction.

There was some evidence to suggest that mentors were most comfortable when dealing with mentees' professional and educational concerns, but were less comfortable when faced with mentees' personal issues. In addition mentors were caused some discomfort by mentees' expectations of their problem-solving powers.

When asked if mentoring had any impact on their professional practice, or on them as individuals, all mentors identified outcomes such as increased skills, greater understanding and greater reflectivity. It could be argued that these outcomes might have been achieved as a result of the training workshops and support groups alone. However, a more likely explanation is that the motivational force provided by the professional fulfilment experienced led to the continued use and development of these skills.

Mentors thought that mentoring would be most effective if it were available to all GPs, based on their assumption that all GPs are under stress. When asked if they would ever consider using the services of a mentor themselves, most said that they would or that they had. Although mentors had no hesitation in saying that everyone should have a mentor, they appeared to suggest that they would not use mentors in the same way as their mentees had. This came across as a wish to make some difference between themselves as mentors, and their mentees.

COMPARING EVALUATION OF MENTORS' PERCEPTIONS WITH THAT OF MENTEES

Widespread support for the mentoring scheme to be extended, improved and made accessible to all was expressed unreservedly by the mentors and mentees interviewed. The reasons offered by both groups were similar in nature, focusing largely on the stressful nature of modern general practice, coupled with the acknowledged reticence of GPs to discuss their problems with each other in the course of normal practice.

Mentors acknowledged the importance of listening skills, and mentees described listening as the most significant and highly rated skill possessed by their mentors. This close match between expectation and reality seemed significant in the mentees' perception of a successful service. Counselling skills were also rated highly and mentees often took personal or stress-related problems to their mentors. There was a mismatch between expectations and reality in this regard, since mentors described being least comfortable when dealing with personal issues. However, it was thought that training and practice, together with sensitivity to gender and culture, could address this problem. There was further divergence of opinion between mentors and mentees in that mentees often expected their mentor to have the power and influence to solve professional problems for them, whereas mentors felt uncomfortable about such expectations. Whilst some mentors wanted to see education as a primary aim of mentoring, mentees felt that they could obtain this service better elsewhere. Likewise they would not consult mentors about clinical matters, considering themselves to be at the same level of expertise as their mentors in this respect.

There was a high level of agreement amongst mentors and mentees that gender and culture were not particularly important. The majority of mentees suggested that professional knowledge and experience were more important, tending to associate this with age and seniority. However, further inquiry in both groups elicited some tentative thoughts about the type of issue which might require a same gender, or same culture, mentor. The sample size in these studies is not large or diverse enough to yield a true picture of the choices mentees would make if they were able.

There was a high level of agreement between mentors and mentees that the time they had invested in mentoring was well spent. For the mentors this feeling resulted from the scheme's perceived success in reducing stress and enhancing job satisfaction. For the mentees, although there were some clearly defined benefits in terms of changes to aspects of their working lives, the main source of their satisfaction was the decrease in their isolation afforded by the opportunity to share their worries and difficulties in a supported and non-judgmental environment.

There was general agreement that modern general practice is characterized by change, role proliferation, greater numbers of patient complaints and a multitude of stresses, leaving the GP ever more vulnerable to stress-related problems. However, there were still worries voiced by both groups about the possibility that stigma might attach to GPs who seek mentors. GPs thought that stigma would be reduced if mentoring were an integral part of the career structure. The suggestion from mentees for reducing stigma was that mentors should also receive mentoring, and mentees should have the opportunity to be mentors simultaneously. There was more support for peer based mentoring from mentees than was expressed by mentors, many of whom felt that professional seniority was relevant in the mentor role. However, the status afforded to the mentor may be in the eyes of the individual mentee rather than in terms of professional status *per se*, and may in part be attributable to mentors receiving special training for the scheme. Since mentors, who themselves have the support of a mentor, are likely to get the best of both worlds, i.e. stress reduction and role satisfaction, the idea that mentor and mentee could be one and the same seems logical.

There were some particular characteristics of the professional community which were significant and needed to be borne in mind when interpreting the results of this evaluation. Most of the GP mentees who participated in the study were lone practitioners subject to varying degrees of professional isolation, or in two 'person' practices, sometimes involving husband/wife or father/son partnerships. There was some evidence that close personal relationships could prevent open communication about certain aspects of professional life. Whereas larger practices may provide a forum for open discussion about problematic issues, the single-handed GP, or those GPs with particularly close relationships within partnerships, might find the provision of an external, objective, professional perspective, such as is offered by a mentor, helpful. In addition, all but two of the GPs we interviewed were Asian and all of the mentors were Asian. Mentoring had particular cultural meaning for the Asian participants, and some of those interviewed told us that they had religious mentors. This familiarity and positive regard for mentoring as a way of meeting personal needs may mean that the GP participants in this study were particularly open to mentoring as a way of meeting professional needs.

All participants enthusiastically co-operated with this evaluation and expressed the view that an evaluation process should be integral to mentoring schemes. Many thought that questionnaires sent to their surgery would not get answered, and that an interview such as the one for this evaluation would be too time consuming to do regularly. Two suggestions were made: centrally devised anonymous feedback forms for mentees and mentors to be activated by the mentor and returned independently; and a published annual report serving to retain mentoring in the professional arena.

Conclusion

Work on this evaluation has led us to make some observations about areas where further research in mentoring might profitably be undertaken. We are conscious that this small scale study in one area is unique in that mentoring schemes have developed in various different ways in other parts of the UK and abroad. A large scale research project could collect information from organizers of schemes, and test participants' perceptions of those schemes by means of independent evaluation. Analysis and comparison of the evaluations would enable commonalities and differences to be described. Such a study could yield information on which mentors' training could be based. Some suggestions for further study are:

- Contrasting funded schemes, such as this one, with unfunded schemes
- Research involving a larger and more diverse population of mentors and mentees to yield a better understanding of the significance of culture and gender
- Exploring comparisons across geographically and locally specific groups
- Comparing GPs who choose not to take part in mentoring schemes with those who do, enabling the issue of non-participation to be examined.

Finally, we are aware that there are potential links between mentoring and other current developments in general practice, such as professional accreditation. Further research in this area could usefully explore the possible impact that linking mentoring schemes with accreditation might have, and the different ways in which this link might be made.

In this chapter we have discussed the application of qualitative methods to a small scale evaluation, and we have given a flavour of the results we obtained. It is our recommendation that others who undertake a similar exercise should consider employing a qualitative framework such as this, which we found in practice to be a highly appropriate approach. The necessary data arose from the participants' exploration of complex themes, in part only emerging as a result of the opportunity for their reflection on complex personal experiences, which was afforded by the evaluation process itself. Without the reflexive dynamic[13] inherent in such an action research model, much of the information would remain inaccessible and unavailable, both to the participants and to the evaluators.

References

1 Eliot T.S. Poem: The Rock, written in 1934. In *Collected Poems 1909–1962*. Faber and Faber, London
2 Kitzinger J.1994 The methodology of focus groups – the importance of interaction between research participants. *Sociology of Health and Illness*, **16**, 103–21
3 Glaser B.G. and Strauss A. 1969 *The Discovery Of Grounded Theory*. Aldine, Chicago, IL.
4 Elliott J. 1991 *Action Research for Educational Change*. Open University Press, Milton Keynes
5 Dadds M. 1993 Thinking and being in teacher action research. In *Reconstructing Teacher Education* (ed. John Elliott). Falmer Press, London
6 Kemmis S. 1989 *Metatheory and Metapractice in Educational Theorizing and Research*. Geelong Deakin University Press, Victoria, Australia
7 For example, the series of articles on qualitative research beginning in the *British Journal of Medicine*, **311**, July 1995, 42–5
8 A fuller account of the evaluation, including the content themes of mentor sessions, is in Chapter 6 of *Mentoring in General Practice* (Freeman R.) included in *Mentoring – The New Panacea?* (ed. Joan Stephenson) 1997. Peter Francis Publishers
9 Howie J.G.R. 1996 Addressing the credibility gap in general practice research. *British Journal of General Practitioners*, **46**(409), 479–81
10 See for example Miles M. and Huberman A. 1994 *An Expanded Sourcebook: Qualitative Data Analysis*. Sage, London
11 See for example Uzzell D. 1995 Ethnographic and action research. In *Research Methods in Psychology* (eds Breakwell G. *et al.*). Sage, London, 302–13
12 Layder D. 1993 *New Strategies in Social Research*. Polity Press, Cambridge
13 Coolican H. 1994 *Research Methods and Statistics in Psychology*. Hodder and Stoughton, London

Creativity and diversity in mentoring: Aspects of personal and professional culture

'There are truths in one country which are falsehoods in another'

(Blaise Pascal)

The concept of holistic mentoring is derived from wider concepts of professional development, all of which embody a Western view of the world. But the two mentor teams who are the major characters in this story had very diverse cultures. The Asian mentor team shared an Eastern view of the world, based on their culture of origin, whilst the team in South West Thames embodied the stereotypical white British culture of the West. The chapter begins by considering the possible effect of culture on the task of mentoring, and explores how the diverse cultures of the two mentor teams influenced their initial perception of the role of the mentor and later, as their work developed, the way in which they set about constructing their identity as GP mentors. Using a theoretical framework of national cultures, the experiences of the two mentor teams are contrasted, not as a measure of implied difference, but in celebration of the diversity of culture, and its capacity to inform and develop understanding.

A further aspect of culture likely to influence thought and action is that of the profession itself, where a collective view of the world prevails, so that perceptions of events and responses to them are influenced by a shared professional culture. Part of the professional culture could be seen as one which encourages a diversity of ideas, so that no single response to perceived need prevails. The second part of the chapter provides an example of such diversity by providing an example of a different helping intervention, which the contributors, for reasons described in their text, refer to as 'co-tutoring'.

Part 1: Importance of culture

Definitions of 'culture' centre on the collective programming of the mind which distinguishes the members of one group of people from another, and leads them to live their lives in ways that are that are shaped by unwritten social codes. A blurred boundary separates an individual's own unique set of personal responses – personality – from those expressions of feeling which, through childhood, are both influenced and modified by the culture of the family, in itself influenced by the wider cultural context of their country of origin. Within the triangle of

the individual, his or her family, and their national culture sit other different layers of culture:

- Ethnic and/or religious level
- Gender
- Generation
- Language
- Social class or caste
- Professional/organizational – the corporate culture of work,

all of which have to be managed alongside each other. Achieving a comfortable fit between the cultural layers is a complex, ongoing task, yet
failure to do so brings an uncomfortable clash of cultures. For myself,
being a woman working in a male dominated profession, brings, at
times, a conflict between feminine and masculine cultures. As a non-
clinician working in general practice, there is the added complication of
being outside of the medical culture, whilst importing into it the cultures
of education and psychology. This at times results in culture clash, when
myself and my colleagues have conflicting perceptions of the same
event, which leads us to very different responses in finding ways of managing it. If there is sufficient elasticity in the personal or organizational
system to tolerate 'other' cultures, and the differing views and perceptions
that arise from them, foreigners are welcomed, they are not always 'understood', but they provide diversity. In the absence of toleration of difference,
there is division and alienation.

How are cultural differences displayed? Hofstede[1] names four aspects of
the manifestations of a culture: symbols, heroes, rituals, and values. Like
the skin of an onion, they are peeled away in layers, with symbols representing the most superficial and values the deepest manifestations, with
heroes and rituals lying in between. From each cultural layer, from religion,
or profession, individual men and women are thrown up to become the
heroes and heroines of the day, people who inspire others in the cultural
group, who can act as role models. Other members of the cultural group
copy their behaviour, and adopt their values.

In medicine, the Hippocratic Oath embodies all four aspects of the profession's cultural manifestation – heroes, symbols, rituals and values.
Hippocrates appears as a founder-hero, the serpent entwined on his
staff becomes the symbol of medical practice, conveying important information to 'outsiders'. This is a powerful symbol of medical culture, one
that is transferred across cultures, recognized and responded to by
people of very different nations. Not very long ago, reciting the Hippocratic
Oath was part of the ritual of admission to the medical profession, a public
declaration of becoming an insider to the profession. Whilst that ritual
aspect of medical culture may have passed, the Oath is still seen as an
embodiment of the values of the profession, values that are continually
referred to and debated. For example, 'I will give no deadly medicine to
anyone if asked, nor suggest any such counsel' is at the centre of ethical
debates on euthanasia, and it is still generally understood that doctors
abstain from the 'seduction of females or males,' although perhaps that
part of the oath concerned with the doctor's undertaking to 'live life

with purity and holiness in order to practise my Art' is more variously interpreted.

Rituals ensure the maintenance of a cultural group, and through them new members gain admission to 'insider knowledge'. All general practitioners can recall the rituals that accompanied their admission as an 'insider' to their (then) new practice, trying to fathom the unwritten codes of the partnership, to glean information about its previous history, working their way in from the edges to find a place for themselves inside the group. Young principals working with their mentors often rehearsed this transitional journey for, although warmly welcomed by their new partners, partnership meetings were sometimes bewildering, as they revealed glimpses of group rituals and beliefs that were never talked about at interview, but were slowly revealed in the process of becoming an insider.

Diversity – cultural issues in mentoring

Differences between cultures are communicated in a number of ways. Some differences are overt, easily seen, and willingly shared with those from outside. Most of us when visiting other countries as a tourist have a deliberate intent to seek out those more superficial differences, delighting in differences in food, pace of life, family life, and organization of the working day.

In the overall context of the mentor meetings, these superficial differences were easily observable. Most of the Asian mentors were first-generation immigrants, and all of them received their medical training overseas, usually in India, their country of origin. This was further strengthened by many years of working experience in British hospital culture, from which was gained postgraduate training and qualification. Whilst all of them were obviously Westernized in dress and language, team meetings gave an opportunity for their first culture to re-assert itself, a time when they could meet together and speak to each other in their own language, and share traditional foods.

The British mentor team behaved similarly, from within their own culture. They too trained in their country of birth, and although team meetings provided the chance to speak to each other informally, the language of their professional culture dominated and only occasionally was personal information exchanged. But food was an equally important part of group ritual; it was described, discussed, and offered with the same level of interest and enthusiasm shown as in the Asian team.

Less discernible, and less accessible to outsiders, are the shared value systems that underpin expressions of a cultural belief, a means of understanding why a cultural group behaves as it does. Unless outsiders seek, or are offered, insights into the cultural norm, they do not have the means to understand the functioning of a cultural group, and the conduct of members remains incomprehensible. The previous chapter commented on the importance of a leader having a good working relationship with their group, and in working with my Asian colleagues I wanted to try, however ineptly, to focus on some of the aspects of cultural harmony and diversity in mentoring. Through exploring the different perceptions that arose, I hoped to develop sufficient insight to catch a glimpse of the deeper layers of cultural values and beliefs which underpin the diversity. Understanding these can produce a more comfortable fit between different layers of culture; desirable, if not essential when working together on a shared project in which so much time and effort has been expended.

This rationale is, of course, in itself culturally biased. My own layers of culture, particularly gender and profession, and my Western view of the world, influence the position that I take up in relation to the mentoring task. An over-riding bias stems from a previous professional culture, psychology, which, like Pandora, is given to opening up forbidden jars. The bias is further extended by my current working culture of professional education, which collectively believes that professional practice is improved, and individual development enhanced, when occasional forays into the deep waters of an individual's inner belief system are made. Such raids upon privacy are justified by the conviction that, handled skilfully (another professional bias) they offer the individual greater insights into how their values and beliefs inform and influence their professional practice, and where they might be in conflict with other people's values (their partner in the practice, for example).

Insight gained in this way can be used to promote understanding, which in turn promotes action for change, in itself an important part of the mentoring process. When working with both mentor teams, I sought opportunities to actively encourage mentors to explore the beliefs and values that underpinned their work and influenced their behaviours. When the two teams came together, the wider understanding and insight gained from these occasions was used for bridge building. The bridge acknowledged cultural difference, without seeking to deny or diminish it, and reached forward to identify and develop shared values – those things which allowed the two teams to work harmoniously on a joint task.

However, additional unforeseen factors accompanied the attempt to build a bridge across diversity, and lurked like the proverbial goblins, waiting to waylay the first traveller attempting to cross. Seeking information about inner beliefs is an uncomfortable process in any culture. When attempts were made to do this, both teams became uneasy, and their unease was heightened by the inevitable clash with the closed defensiveness of their medical culture. At times, my personal courage to persist in the exploration failed; it was more comfortable to adopt the dominant professional culture and settle for discussing superficialities.

Again, discussing cultural diversity with Asian mentors who live and work in the UK risked opening a divide. Asking questions about their culture implied their continuing different identity, pushing them back into 'Indian-ness' when they had striven hard for a measure of English-ness, the right of entry to a British cultural group, and acceptance of their right to belong. Private conversations with mentors showed how the painful injustices of racism have underscored efforts to integrate with, and become accepted by, British medical colleagues and be viewed as equals. And culturally, at times, they were also puzzled by my apparent need to analyse and explore a process which was internal to them, which did not absorb them, as it did me, so that in the process I was the one to be set apart as the outsider.

Only as the mentors began to trust my own essential belief in them, and I thereby became slightly more confident and hopefully less clumsy in framing questions, were we at times able to talk together of cultural values and beliefs, and lay down the first planks of the bridge, even if somewhat precariously. When this state was achieved, the two mentor teams came together for a joint workshop, hoping that it would provide further opportunities for glimpsing the deeper layers of each other's culture through sharing a task. Mentors paired off across the teams, and spoke privately to each other about their experience of mentoring, then worked together in plenary sessions, before sharing a formal dinner at the end of the day.

Evaluating this event, the Asian mentors spoke warmly of their feelings of inclusion; many said it was the first time that they had felt themselves accepted as equals, of being welcomed and 'drawn in'. The British team were humbled, both by the contrast in the professional working conditions and by the greater insight (as they saw it) of their Asian colleagues into the complexity of mentoring, a deeper level of insight which, they said, they themselves gained through working alongside them in the workshop.

On this and other occasions, the deeper layers of culture were glimpsed and made visible, but for the most part they remained hidden; not exactly invisible, but unspoken. After the shared workshop, some of the mentors in the South team pondered over the indefinable aspect of difference that so many of them envied:

'what *is* it about them [the Asian mentors] . . . they have this sort of "inner" quality . . . they seem to be much more at home with living inside themselves somehow . . .'

whilst another mentor said with some exasperation:

'I don't know exactly what it is they've got . . . tranquillity? Whatever it is, I want some of it!'

What was the nature of this difference? I suspect it can never be fully explained, but further thoughts about cultural diversity can be found in work which explores national culture.

Four dimensions of culture

Equally frustrated by trying to define the nature of difference, and impatient with the vagueness of what represents national culture, Hofstede[2] set about conducting a large-scale survey of forty independent nations. From this he defined four dimensions of culture. Each of the national cultures he then ranked high or low on the four dimensions, to provide a more distinctive cultural profile. His survey was repeated after 4 years, remained stable, and has become one of the key indicators of cultural meaning. The four dimensions are individualism, power–distance, uncertainty avoidance, and gender. A summary of each of these dimensions is followed by an attempt to apply the experience of the mentor teams as they set about defining their mentor role with his theory of national culture. This is an ambitious attempt. Without wishing to sound defensive, it is in part constrained by the paucity of literature in general practice about how the doctor's *own* culture influences their perception of their task – most writings concentrate on the attitudes of patients from other cultures. If there are authors out there who have all the answers, I apologize in advance that my search failed to locate you!

INDIVIDUALISM

Individualism is the degree to which a culture encourages individual as opposed to *collectivist*, or group-centred, concerns. It is drawn from the broader framework of social psychology, which develops concepts based on key differences between members of individual and collectivist societies.

In this dimension, the differences of culture start from a consideration of the differing perspectives of Western and Eastern society. Eastern and African societies usually fall into the category of a collectivist society; British, American and European into individualistic. The holistic model of mentoring intervention belongs to individualism. It is based on a belief in the rightness of self-development, the right of individuals to self-actualize, to pursue their desired aims towards self-fulfilment. It assumes that this is what mentees, in their various ways, want for themselves.

But the concept of 'self' is a peculiarly Western view. Once, when working in Hong Kong, and discussing self-development with a group of Chinese doctors, we discovered that there are no words in either Cantonese or Mandarin which translate into the idea of 'doing your own thing'; they simply do not exist. Writing of Chinese culture, Bond[3] explains why.

'the social orientation of the Chinese is reflected in the higher endorsement they give to group-related traits and roles, as well as the fact that their ideal self is closely involved in social relationships. The dimensions they use to perceive themselves and others are likewise focused on interpersonal concerns, not on mastery of the external world or absorption with narrowly personal processes' (p. 34).

Hence, in an *individualistic* society, identity is based on the individual, who is encouraged to seek independence from the family group, and indeed is viewed as immature if they fail to do so at the appropriate time. Children are taught to think in terms of 'I' rather than 'we', to 'stand up for themselves'. As young adults, they are encouraged to 'do their own thing', to follow their own ambitions and desires, to continue to 'speak their mind' and assert themselves. This enables them to fulfil the expectation that as adults they will look after themselves, and maximize opportunities which progress their status. The focus is on personal initiative and achievement. Education increases both earning power, which is distributed at the discretion of the earner, and status, leading to increased self-respect and feelings of self-worth. Employment is based on merit and possession of requisite skills and knowledge. Disharmony is tolerated. Privacy is seen as a right; the desired state is individual freedom.

By contrast, a *collectivist* society is characterized by membership of an extended family group, overarched by kith and kin. This group is the primary source of loyalty and allegiance. Individual identity is based in membership of family groups; it is the network to which one belongs which both advances your interests and protects your wellbeing. Achievements are seen as individual gains, but ones which benefit the extended family group. The cost of educational opportunity is shared between an entire family group. Any benefit this brings to the student, including higher professional earnings, are distributed amongst the family as a shared benefit.

Employment is offered via family networks, and takes into account the position of the employees' 'ingroup'. Employers – the superior few – have the responsibility of finding a task in the workplace for members of the extended family. Unemployed or elderly members of the group are supported and cared for by those who are employed. The shame and humiliation of transgressing laws and social codes are felt collectively; the group, not only the individual, loses face. Living in harmony, without confrontation, is the desired state.

Theory applied to mentoring: the two mentor teams
The Asian mentor team could realistically be seen as straddling the collectivist–individualist divide, coming originally from the former, yet making their later life in the latter. Yet, at times there were glimpses of collectivism. From the start of the project, the identity of the Asian mentor team as a group functioning within a close, extended network was obvious; it felt like an extended family. The team told me very early on that their Educational Director, although white like myself, had spent his childhood in India, and therefore he 'knew their ways' – he was part of the network, a member of the family. By this was meant he shared their collectivist values, and this was obvious in his professional work, as well as in his family life. The professional commitment of mentoring, of coming to the support groups and shared workshops, carrying out the accompanying administrative procedures, was adopted wholeheartedly; they were collectively conscientious about fulfilling the project requirements. They were also proud of their mentor role, and owned it in their professional community.

There were occasions too in this team when their strong allegiance to their family group over-rode competing professional demands. At times I was told that individual mentors had to 'return to the old place' at very short notice because of illness in their family, or some family crisis arose which required the attendance of the entire family group to resolve.

On these occasions, absences from the team – even when the absence of a mentor involved some disruption to the meeting – were simply accounted for: 'he has gone home'. The rest was surmised. The sudden lengthy absences from their practice (and some were single-handed practitioners) seemed to lack the loud accompanying trauma experienced by doctors elsewhere when they have to suddenly disappear from their surgeries, and this seemed in part due to the fact that friends and family members from the extended network quickly moved in to maintain a service to patients. Members of the mentor team were clearly involved with each other; a strong sense of membership existed, which for some extended to include regular meetings between mentor members and their spouses.

The South team had to make more deliberate and obvious attempts to unite as a team. They had to seek a comfortable compromise between their own individuality and the necessary collective identity which would enjoin them to the mentoring task. The introductory workshops brought a superficial adherence to a collective view as to what the action of a mentor might be, and the values that underpinned the mentoring task. This gained admittance to an organizational group, the mentor team. Once inside, company rules could be reviewed, re-written, adapted, or ignored. During that process three mentors kept firmly to their individualistic culture, saying that whilst they upheld the concept of mentoring being developed, they preferred to stay outside of the team and 'do their own thing'. This was acted out by not attending the support groups (which had been seen as a prerequisite for developing mentor skills and knowledge – a company rule) and failing to provide records of their mentor interviews.

There was little obvious evidence in this team of personal relationships going beyond the shared support for each other in carrying out the task – they clearly enjoyed working with each other, and used the opportunity for some informal networking, but this did not go beyond professional life.

POWER–DISTANCE

Power–distance relates to how far a culture encourages the exertion of power. In high power–distance countries (of which India is one), power is a basic fact of life; its legitimacy is irrelevant, those with power are expected to act powerfully and not trust others. Inequality is accepted; everyone has their rightful place, subordinates do not disagree or question their lot. In low power–distance countries (Britain ranks as low–medium) inequalities are minimized; there is a preference for those with power to act less powerful than they are. The ideal workplace is one where employees are consulted before decisions are made, the relationship between the boss and subordinates is one of colleagues, and employees are not afraid to disagree.

Application to mentoring
The influence of power–distance on the development of a mentor-identity was most clearly seen at the beginning of the mentor project. In both teams, at the start of the introductory workshops, a brainstorming exercise was used to uncover participants' own definitions of a mentor. This exercise gave the first visible evidence of diversity between the two cultures in their perceptions of power and authority, and was likely to influence not only how they defined the mentor role, but how they saw themselves acting within it. These are the dominant words used in conjunction with definitions of a mentor, placed within the two cultures of East (represented by the Asian team) and West (the white, British team).

East	West
Guru	Facilitator
Master	Equal peer
Role model	Supporter
Teacher	Adviser

Overall, the Asian team *sought* authority; they perceived mentors to be authority figures, receiving respect on the basis of greater knowledge, wisdom, and expertise. They did not shrink from claiming this element of authority for themselves, as potential mentors, without in any way seeking self-aggrandizement. The qualities of a guru include possession of an extra dimension of knowledge, greater mastery of an art, and charisma which induces others to follow. These were the qualities associated with the role by their potential mentees, without which mentors would not be afforded the proper respect conversant with the role. As previous chapters show, the Asian team moved away from this more traditional notion of a mentor, skilfully incorporating the concept of facilitation, but it is also important to remember that this Western view of the mentor's role was at times a disappointment to their Asian mentees, who wanted a guru, a master who would 'fix' things for them.

India scored high on Hofstede's power–distance ranking. Allowing for the variable of the Asian team's dual nationality, it does seem as if these mentors were quite comfortable with the idea of having power, perhaps because their culture is based in an acceptance of inequality.

By contrast, the British team *avoided* the element of authority, perceiving mentors as facilitators of the mentee's development. Authority came from greater experience, not greater knowledge, and was seen as indirect, distant from the mentoring process. Britain has a low-medium score on this dimension; the mentors were keen to stress the equality of their position – the mentor as an equal, supportive peer. The focus was on the mentor's facilitating, encouraging role, and anxiety was expressed that they might be as 'experts'. Nonetheless, they did share with gurus the desire to be an inspiration to others.

Power–distance in learning and teaching
For me, one of the many delightful aspects of Eastern culture is that it places teachers amongst highly respected authority figures, not to be questioned or disagreed with. I much enjoy occupying this safe place, even if only transiently! And, as their team leader, the Asian mentors afforded me unquestioning respect for my authority as their designated leader and teacher. This is paradoxical to the Western style of postgraduate education, in which the teacher sets up a dialogue with students, seeking the contribution of their experience, ideas and thoughts, courting disagreement as a critical evaluation of the subject being taught and, as a consequence, offering up their authority as a teacher for the students' scrutiny.

At the beginning of the workshop, I spoke with the Asian team about this difference, and stressed that, as I was learning too about the whole process of mentoring in general practice, everything I offered was open to critical review. I attempted to disown any authority, encouraging them to suspend their cultural politeness, and enter into questioning discussion.

Initially, it did not happen. Participants spoke animatedly amongst themselves, but addressed few questions to me. When I spoke there was silence, and it was apparent that I had their full attention. In one of our earliest meetings, I was relieved to be interrupted in mid-sentence by a dominant group member. The relief was short lived, as he was quickly hushed into silence by his peers. In the tea break the group's 'elder statesman' came and apologized for his colleague's 'disrespect'. For a while, then, it seemed that suspending the cultural norm was uncomfortable; it did not easily fit, although as my working relationship with this team became more established, we quickly encountered the opposite problem, when at times I struggled to be heard above the team's lively and animated discourse.

This questioning of authority is a frequent source of culture clash, when layers of culture struggle to accommodate each other, as this discussion with a primary school teacher from a school in North London, with a mix of ethnic children illustrates:

'once, at an open evening, I said to the Sikh parents of a boy who had recently entered the school that he was very quiet, and did not say much. His father said that is the way he is brought up. I then said that he was an intelligent boy, and that I was encouraging him to speak up, to join answering questions, in effect – to make more noise. And the child's mother then said quietly – yes – he is behaving in this way at home. Then the father told me quite angrily that his son's noisy behaviour at home had caused his own father, who lived with the family, to take him to task, saying that he should take the child in hand, and take him to the temple more often. Inadvertently, I had caused this father to be criticised by his family, for not disciplining the child enough, for not bringing him up in the "right way".'[4]

Here was a child learning to live between two cultures – to be one person at school, another at home. Both he and his father had to manage the misfit between the cultural layer of generations, when the elders of the family were present, who considered it undesirable for children to be curious, noisy learners, and desirable for a father to be a strict disciplinarian.

UNCERTAINTY AVOIDANCE

Uncertainty avoidance relates to levels of tolerance of uncertainty, or, as Pugh[5] describes it, the 'ease with which the culture copes with novelty' (p. 77). High uncertainty avoidance cultures need clarity and order; they are threatened by uncertainty, experiencing stress and anxiety as a result. This is avoided by strong rules which maintain order; there is low tolerance of deviation from the norm: work hard, don't break the rules, and you've got a job for life is the philosophy, whereas in low uncertainty avoidance cultures they regard uncertainty as a part of life: each day is taken as it comes, and a more pragmatic view of rules is taken. Employees expect to work for firms for much shorter periods.

Application to mentoring
From this dimension of culture emerged two themes – the mentor team's relationship to me as the 'teacher' facilitator in the early workshops, and

their individual experiences of uncertainty in the process of mentoring work.

There was diversity between the two teams in their response to my role as the workshop leader. Hofstede[6] comments relevantly on this aspect when describing his observational study of an International Teachers Programme, which recruited postgraduate students from a number of countries. He correlated his second cultural dimension of uncertainty avoidance with the preferred learning styles of the participants. Asian countries were ranked amongst those whose tolerance of uncertainty was poor; countries where rules and structure were highly valued. Students from these countries expected their teachers to be experts, and to know all the answers. The process of learning was a search for the one, correct answer, and increased respect was afforded to teachers who spoke, or wrote, in obscure academic language.

A previous teaching experience in the far East had thrown up all of these aspects, and had alerted me to the subsequent difficulty of making a reasonable assessment about how much of the teaching is understood, and can be usefully reflected upon before applying it relevantly. Although this in itself is a Western perception of the necessary conditions for effective learning, it did seem a prerequisite for developing effective mentoring.

For the Asian team, in the implementation phase of our meetings, when my authority as teacher was unquestioned, they at first looked to me to tell them how to proceed, to give the right answer, spurning the Western way of discovery learning. There were some visible signs of dismay when I at times admitted that I did not know the answer. And, this produced an uncomfortable culture clash at times, as they searched for answers from the authority source, and I strove to avoid giving answers, wanting them to develop their own ideas through exploration; they told me afterwards that this nearly drove them mad! Yet later, as the support groups became established, the Asian mentors became far more adept in the art of reflecting on practice, exploring in depth their individual understanding of concepts, than their Western counterparts. It was this aspect that gave rise to the comment quoted at the start of this chapter, when the South team became aware of the Asian team's power of reflective insight.

The British team came from a country designated by Hofstede as one which could tolerate uncertainty, and as such were likely to despise too much structure, represented in items such as course programmes, and prefer open-ended learning situations in which they themselves sought 'answers'. Certainly the group saw learning to become a mentor as being in itself an education; they were comfortable with the absence of 'answers' and viewed my presence as one which resourced their learning. Participants needed little encouragement to interact with ideas and concepts, to state their own position and thinking. They were not that keen on teacher-authority either, and certainly academic language did not increase respect, for the team made clear their impatience with what they heard as 'educational jargon' or 'psychological claptrap'. Only when unfamiliar concepts were constructed in familiar language and terms, and clearly seen as relevant to the mentoring task, did it appear to increase respect for the teacher's knowledge, and then only marginally.

Uncertainty avoidance in the mentoring process

For both teams, a major focus relating to the cultural dimension of tolerating anxiety was the learning theme discussed in the previous chapter, that of becoming constructively challenging. Although the necessity of balancing support for one's mentee with appropriate challenge was not denied, envisaging oneself doing it was another matter.

Here the different layers of culture immediately presented themselves. The two teams were united in sharing the constraints of their professional culture. Doctors are well versed in the art of avoiding discussion about, and investigation of, causes of conflict between practitioners, the profession as a whole preferring the Eastern way of presenting to the world a harmonious face. It is legitimate as a doctor to confront patients with unhealthy lifestyles, to seize opportunities in the consultation to promote healthier living, but directly confronting peers with their unhealthy professional relationships is avoided. This made it hard for the mentors to anticipate developing and using skills for positive confrontation, for neither team had within their different cultures the experience of confrontation and challenge.

However, the nature of the conflict experienced by the mentees showed the diversity of power–distance between the two cultures. In the Asian team, mentors were working with Asian mentees who had high on their agenda their conflict with higher authority figures from their regional health authority. The source of conflict was commonly about money, about insufficient funding being given to improve practice premises, or employ extra staff. There was conflict too with those in authority on the local education board. This panel of doctors made decisions on the dispersal of funds which paid for doctors to pursue their continuing education, reimbursing the cost of employing locum cover, as well as paying course fees.

The Asian team struggled with these mentees. It was said earlier in this chapter that, whilst the mentor team moved from a cultural view of mentors as masters, some of their mentees had not. These mentees looked towards their mentor to use their own authority to intervene, and settle the conflict in their favour. They did not expect an equal world, and uncertainty could be countered by the intervention of your own superior approaching those superiors who held power through funds. You used the network to ensure a good outcome. And the mentors, caught between cultures, naturally at first contemplated taking on the confrontations on behalf of the mentees, before moving towards developing strategies which helped the mentees confront these problems themselves.

Conflict was on the agenda of many of the white, Western mentees coming to the British team – but their conflict was with their partners in the group practice. Although it showed the same theme of power and equality, frequently the source of conflict was about money, and their own share of partnership profits. They were angry about the apparent unequal distribution of work amongst partners, and sought clearer evidence of equality in the workplace. But these mentees expected their mentors to advise them about how to proceed, to help them devise strategies which might improve their working relationships. They did not expect their mentor to directly intervene in what was, to them, a dispute between colleagues; indeed it is difficult to imagine a scenario where a mentor presents himself to a group practice demanding justice on behalf of his mentee!

These culturally bound, conflicting values make it difficult for people to anticipate their behaviour in a new situation, and when this happens they say that they know they 'ought' but they 'can't'. This conflict of values was particularly well illustrated in one of the Asian mentor meetings, at a time when the mentors had become well established in their work:

S [the mentor] tells of his struggle with a rude, angry, embittered mentee whose current agenda was to coerce his mentor into acting to restore his status. S had told his mentee that he would speak to the appropriate authority, but could not ensure his success, whereupon he was shown the door by the mentee in no un- certain way. But then the mentee had telephoned and asked to see him again, leaving S uncertain about what he should do. From the following discussion, it was clear that the mentor sought permission to give up on this abusive mentee. The group disagreed, pointing out that the canker of resentment and anger was 'eating away' at this mentee, its repression was affecting his health, and the mentor needed to 'go back in there'. Looking distinctly apprehensive, the mentor asked what it was he must go back in to do – he could not envisage what task he might engage in. The group constructed an opening script to help the mentor bring about a cathartic discussion, in which the mentee could be encouraged to offload reasons for his anger.

S smiled urbanely, but looked uncomfortable with the idea of getting beneath the surface, questioning the group's conviction that the mentee would only move for- ward if he were helped to face his own negative attitude. The group then became very supportive to S, arranging for one of them to ring him after he had seen his difficult mentee, so that he could offload his own feelings about how he managed to confront the anger.

This session presented the mentor with a conflict of values. It was not the way of Eastern culture to confront anger so directly; it was preferable to maintain harmony. Even when faced with his peers' certainty that it was the 'right thing to do', it was difficult for the mentor to think himself into the confronting role. This, in addition to tolerating the uncertainty of the outcome, moved him more firmly into his own culture of origin.

For the British mentors, the conflict of values was represented differ- ently, through the process of sharing their work. As the previous illustra- tion shows, the Asian mentors entered the process of their mentor support groups with nothing short of gusto. It appeared as if the idea of reflecting on their actions as mentors, analysing their response to their mentees, and having space to tell their story, was familiar practice. Was this in part due to the mentors' collective identity in their network, so that they behaved as would an extended family, speaking freely and animatedly with each other?

The individualist nature of national British culture perhaps contributes to more guarded, cautious sharing of experience. Enforcing this is another layer of culture, that of profession, stemming from the isolated, private nature of general practice, where the patient is seen behind closed doors, with only the occasional presence of a trainee GP to observe the practitioner at work; a very private enterprise indeed.

When given space to share the details of one's own mentoring practice, the potential conflict of values can be a contributing factor which makes it difficult to start. As the previous chapter discussed, mentors in the British team resisted going into the detail about their mentoring role, taking the option of a quick skim past the process of the mentoring meeting. When challenged about superficiality, they protested that they must protect the confidentiality of their mentee. This professional value, so obviously honourable, and therefore so difficult to question, disguised the fact that they were protecting themselves from bringing their work for the scrutiny of their peers. It was they as mentors being discussed, not their mentees, and it was this conflict of values that the reflective format was designed to address. The format was never used in the Asian team, for it was never needed.

But this is not to suggest that the Asian team dealt more easily with deeper, more personal areas on their mentees' agendas. Indeed there was a clear divergence between the two teams when it came to responding to more personal issues in mentoring, such as family problems, or marital disharmony. On these occasions, the Asian mentors were far less comfortable. Again, their collective view supported the theoretical need for mentors to allow mentees to rehearse hindrances to their professional development, but they were uncomfortable with doing so.

Conversely, mentors in the British team described marital and family pressures which added to the stress of their mentee. Although they were clear that the mentor role was not that of a therapist, in their support groups they at times explored psychodynamic frameworks to increase their understanding of how conflicting family roles heightened stress. And, at these times, some mentors were prepared to share with each other how these related to their own life situations.

MASCULINITY AND FEMININITY

In this last dimension, gender is represented as a national cultural dimension. In masculine cultures (for example Australia) performance is what counts: big and fast are beautiful, machismo is essential, ambition the driving force. Sex roles are clearly differentiated; men should be assertive and dominating. A show of strength is the response to conflicts: governments spend more on arms and less on economic aid to poorer countries. Liberating women is interpreted as appointing them to jobs previously held by men. Few women are in positions of power, or hold political posts. In feminine cultures, small and slow are beautiful; sex roles are complementary and less differentiated, so that men also take on caring and nurturing roles. Governments spend less on arms and more on the environment, and assisting other poorer countries, as well as providing a welfare state. More women hold political positions. Sweden is commonly cited as an example of a feminine culture.

Whilst this dimension is interesting to consider in relation to mentoring, applying the framework is constrained by the scheme's limited experience of male and female cultures in the development of mentoring. In this final part of the discussion on culture, the application of the gender dimension moves between mentoring and the professional, organizational culture of medicine.

Application to mentoring
By virtue of the fact that male mentors take on nurturing caring roles, does that steer mentoring towards a feminine culture, a cultural subgroup operating within the larger confines of the masculine culture of medicine? But, if this were so, how do we explain the absence of a significant number of women in both mentor teams – the Asian team of ten mentors includes only one woman, and in the South team, there are four women in a team of 17.

This is very different representation from mentoring programmes run in the NHS, many of which are run by women and are set in the wider context of equal opportunity. These mentor projects are designed to actively encourage and support women to get into senior management and become consultants. Their objective is to help women take charge of their own career, maximizing opportunities for their professional development, based on the assumption (well supported by evidence) that women doctors have unique difficulties when working within the unpredictable, difficult, macho, masculine culture of the NHS. Some of these hospital-based mentoring programmes are run by women, exclusively for women. These programmes perceive mentors as compensatory to the power of patronage. Mentors, working through the appraisal system to offer career advice and ideas on professional development, are a further means of empowering women, helping them to realize their potential, and get to the top.

At the time of writing, the representation of women amongst current mentees is around 38%. There are plenty of variables which could explain this, and of course the percentage fluctuates over time. Apart from the conventional professional gender issues, like balancing child care with practice commitments, or seeing all the female patients with gynaecological problems, do women general practitioners feel themselves to be in a more equal position with their male partners in practice than their colleagues in secondary care? When compared with hospital medicine, does the relative absence of a hierarchical career structure mean that women general practitioners can get where they want, without particular let or hindrance from the masculine culture? It is known that in hospital medicine the career structure, and the way in which careers were organized, prevented many women from realizing their potential. Does general practice present women with fewer obstacles to fulfilment?

It is tempting to say that, within the limitations of this relatively small mentor scheme, it would appear so. Women mentees in the scheme are always asked if they would prefer to have a woman mentor; all of them so far have said they simply do not mind – as the external evaluation of the model showed, the skills of the mentor were far more important to mentees than their gender or culture. The agendas women take to their mentors did not appear to be severely weighted towards discussing the inequalities that their female identity has brought about. Although there was occasional evidence from some women mentees of the bullying behaviours of their male partners (an aspect discussed in Chapter 6 by Neil Munro from his viewpoint as a mentor), male mentees also indicated that, at times, they felt themselves to be victims of their partners' aggressive and dominating attitudes (some of whom, it could be assumed, were women). On the whole, looking at the data from the mentor scheme, women practitioners seem to share with their male colleagues very similar issues about professional development, and balancing work with home life.

But this last aspect, a regular inclusion in the working agenda of mentees, provides a more concrete example of an organizational aspect of gender found in both primary and secondary work settings. It is in this area, of establishing work patterns, that women can be seen as blazing the trail for men, making a gender-based issue important to men as well as women. Allen's extensive study[7] found that

'many of the problems and constraints encountered by women doctors in developing their careers were exactly the same for men' (p. 237)

and one of the constraints encountered by women meant that they perforce led the way in establishing flexible working patterns that balance family life with work.

Whilst maintaining family life is in itself a major task, there are many reasons for working part-time, not all of them children. Perhaps it was, when observing women, men could not help but notice that creative energy and enthusiasm for the professional task is increased by spending time away from it. More male doctors wish to negotiate for themselves flexible working patterns, to become job-sharers, or have a part-time practice commitment, to make space for other activities, clinical and non-clinical, which serve as a replenishment of interest and energy. And increasingly, this flexibility is seen as an important part of recruitment and retention of an expensively trained workforce in medicine.

The desire of both men and women in medicine for more flexible working has begun a challenge to the organizational culture of medicine. To allow a culture to change, a critical mass has to be achieved. As 50% of doctors in training are now women, there is a stronger chance that a sufficiently critical mass will be achieved, and bring about a more representative leadership in medicine which can set about deconstructing the shibboleths of its masculine culture.

When male mentors from both teams were interviewed, to find out more about their identification with the role, part of their motivation for doing the job stemmed from the stimulus that this different activity brought to their professional life. Perhaps few women see becoming a mentor in this light. Finding out more about the influence of gender on the mentoring task is one of many future research questions for the developing scheme.

Conclusion

The paucity of available literature on cultural issues in the mentoring relationship means that the observations and experiences described in this chapter can be seen primarily as prompts to further thinking and debate. It is difficult to write and talk about culture, which is presumably why so few people do, possibly because it incurs the risk of being berated for racism, when seeing the world differently implies value judgements about the superiority of one group over another.

Working with two different mentor teams confronted us all with the need to think more carefully about cultural issues in mentoring relationships, and in my leadership function with both teams. It was a need for which both teams are profoundly grateful, as the opportunity to learn diverse and different things from each other about mentoring, and professional life, continues to provide a highly valued source of learning.

At the end of the day, we found more factors that united the diverse cultures in the project work, and brought about similar outcomes. As the external evaluators told us in Chapter 7, the skills of the mentor to be receptive, compassionate, and challenging in their work were seen by mentees as being far more important than race, culture, or gender. This finding is supported in the literature,[8] in the same way that when doctors are judged by their ethnic patients on the treatment which they give, the doctor's nationality appears as a secondary issue.[9] So our experience thus far suggests that doctors working in vastly different circumstances, coming from opposite cultures, and having very different life experiences, can develop requisite mentor skills, and put them to good effect.

But this begs the question as to whether a Western model of intervention is appropriate when the recipients of it are rooted in other cultures. We have no right to impose our Western individualistic culture on others, particularly when, as the South team mentors found, we have still ourselves much to learn from the cultures of the East. Some mentors are now working with junior doctors from abroad who, once their training is completed, will return to their country of origin. These mentees might be much more comfortable with, and would make better use of, an intervention which is more closely aligned to their own collectivist culture.

Second-generation immigrant doctors, like the Asian mentors, are more culturally flexible; they too have had to become adept at straddling cultures. But, in the privacy of the mentoring relationship, they might wish to discuss the conflict of values that this living between cultures brings, and they can only do that when their own culture of origin is not ignored, but explored, and included as a real and diverse dimension of their personality. Supposing this is so, can it be successfully undertaken only by mentors who share the same cultural background? This in itself has implications for future recruitment of mentors. It is apparent that, as mentoring develops in general practice, the effect of culture on the mentoring relationship becomes a further rich area for research and exploration.

Part 2: Diversity – an aspect of professional culture

In the first half of this chapter, aspects of personal culture were discussed to show that whilst the qualities of an effective mentor have been seen to override race and gender, the culture of origin influences the perception of a given role and its purpose.

Professional culture also influences perceptions. Part of the culture of general practice is to celebrate difference, and creating programmes to foster the continuing education and improvement of the practitioner is no exception. Increasingly, course organizers and GP tutors in general practice are experimenting with more informal helping interventions, which aim to offer some form of support to their peers, even if transiently. The following contribution, although using a fictitious scenario, is intended to provide one such example of professional diversity.

Co-tutoring in general practice
The East Anglian Co-tutoring Team

Co-tutoring is a process whereby a pair or trio of peers (usually general practitioners) meet on a regular basis. In each session, time is divided so that each person has a turn to talk and think through problems or issues of concern to them. The principle is that the listener, with an attitude of respect and acceptance, allows the speaker to air their thoughts, develop their own agenda, identify desired outcomes and work out a means of achieving them. The listener and the speaker develop particular skills to facilitate this process. The underlying belief is that with good attention, active listening and support, individuals are empowered to sort out and solve their own problems. They become more effective professionally and are able to identify some of their learning needs.

Whenever we have run workshops to describe co-tutoring, we avoid lecturing as far as possible. Instead, we encourage people to participate actively, i.e. to practise and rehearse skills, after which we try and answer questions and generate discussion on what they have experienced. We propose to structure our part in this chapter in a similar way. First we offer a fictional scenario of a 'typical' co-tutoring session to give an idea how we work. Then we attempt to answer some of the questions which this vignette might pose for you. In this way we hope to:

- Describe some of the theoretical basis for co-tutoring
- Explain why we think it is so valuable
- Consider how people might learn how to become good co-tutors
- Describe our own experience with it
- Try and answer potential criticisms of the method.

A CO-TUTORING SCENARIO

One evening at 8 pm. The two GPs meeting are Iain and Helen. They have been meeting every month over the last year.

They start with sharing something that that has gone well or is new/ good since their last meeting. They each, with encouragement from the other, think of three positive things. They agree who is going to start as speaker and for how long. They decide on 20 minutes each with time for feedback at the end in order to finish at 9 pm.

Helen goes first. Iain sits and listens attentively.

Helen: Well I want to carry on with my ideas for my audit that I talked about last time. I found it really helpful to think through my ideas on HRT use. I am clear about the criteria I want to use, although I want to get the partners to help me with the actual standards.

Iain: Mmm . . . sounds good . . . so you want to carry on with your ideas . . .

Helen: I know what I want to do, it is the 'how' really . . . What I don't know is how I can get an agreement on the standards and collect the information.

Iain: So do you want to look at the agreement first? Tell me what's hard about it?

Helen: Well, discussing it at a meeting is likely to be difficult, that is if I can get it on the agenda! The real problem is persuading David [practice manager] to put it down for our next practice meeting. He tends to be quite firm about focusing on financial matters to the exclusion of other topics. The problem is that we don't all meet at any other time so audit has to be dealt with at these meetings. His idea of audit and mine are very different . . . he wants audit to look for ways of making money for the practice . . . as does Jim [senior partner] come to think of it. (She pauses, looking thoughtful, and after a while looks directly at Iain).

Iain: That's helpful to be aware of; so you say you need to persuade David first . . .

Helen: Yes – yes that's the problem! He's really difficult. I don't think he respects me . . . a mere woman doctor! Actually he really makes me angry, he's so patronizing.

Iain: . . . that sounds really difficult for you . . .

Helen: Yes when he talks to me I feel as if my ideas are a waste of time. I'm sure that my last project failed because of his negativity . . . it must have affected the staff . . . and they were the ones who were collecting the information . . . actually I'm still quite angry about that time . . . I suppose David is the key person to get on my side for both of the problems.

Iain: That makes sense . . . OK . . . so how are you going to do that?

Helen: Well my audit idea is really good . . . I know it will be worthwhile; it was so helpful thinking it out last time. So I'm not going to be put off by David . . . for goodness sake I am a partner!

But I do want to do it . . . and I need people on my side. So perhaps I could find some time to chat with David . . . I think it would be helpful to understand his views on clinical audit . . . I've no idea what he really thinks about it . . . it would be good to involve him . . . and ask for his suggestions. I could also chat separately with the other partners and tell them about my ideas . . . and ask for their help in thinking through the audit. Yes I feel good about that.

Iain: Well done. When might you be able to do this?

Helen: Well I need to find a good time to meet David . . . not when he is doing the payroll! He's always in a foul mood when that happens. In fact when I think about it most of my chats have been when either one or both of us have been in the middle of doing something else . . . you know what it's like . . . we bump into each other in the office, or in the corridor . . . hopeless really . . . no wonder we don't communicate well at times. What I must do is to fix a time to meet with him in his room when we both have some space . . . yes . . . I can do that soon. As for the others, I usually meet up at coffee time, so I can see them all . . . over the next week.

They finish off with feedback:

Helen: What did you do well as a listener, Iain?

Iain: Well, I did listen well. At the beginning I paused for a long time while you were thinking about your agenda and gave you time to come up with the standards and the information collecting.

Helen: Yes, I agree you listened really well . . . and what was particularly helpful to me was that you accepted my ideas . . . when David blocks my ideas I start to question how good I am . . . What else? . . . Yes, I found it really helpful when you asked me to think when I would put my ideas into practice.

Iain: I was aware that when you expressed your anger about David I didn't really pick it up but moved on to help you think about your next steps. Would you have liked me to have done anything more about it?

Helen: No! . . . Well that's not true really . . . I find anger so difficult that I avoid it. I suppose it might have been helpful but I am always ashamed of my anger and how others might react . . . and how you might . . .

Iain: It would be fine with me . . . what do you think would have helped? I would be happy to help you deal with your anger more.

Helen: Well this has already helped just talking about it. I would feel safer to talk it through more on another occasion, thanks.

Iain: Anything else that you would have liked from me?

Helen: No . . . thanks, that was very useful.

At this point, after the feedback, the two doctors would then swap roles, so that Helen would listen to Iain, using the same process of listening.

THE CO-TUTORING PROCESS

This fictitious example represents a reasonably 'typical' co-tutoring session. We offer participants some guidelines for co-tutoring and Helen and Iain largely followed them. The nub of what they were doing was to listen actively to each other so that each could understand the main issues for themselves and find their own ways forward. In the first session Helen had a prepared agenda. She knew what she wanted to achieve but didn't know how. With Iain's prompting she identified some blocks and also some strategies for overcoming them. Iain helped her focus on an action plan in order to achieve her objectives. After that they would have changed roles, with Helen listening to Iain, and in both cases would have finished with feedback. This gives the listener a chance to reflect on the co-tutoring process, rather than the content, and perhaps take away ideas for subsequent sessions.

Participants in our co-tutoring programme particularly welcome the opportunity to be listened to and the support which co-tutoring gives. The process of being listened to also helps clarify the issues and the desired course of action. Things fall into place as they are being talked about, which aids the whole process of reflection. This is as applicable to interpersonal and emotional matters as it is to practical action. Some participants have been able to make action plans as a result of co-tutoring. These relate to tasks to be undertaken in order to reach a specific goal in the practice (as with Helen) or they might take the form of personal learning plans. Sharing an action plan with another person and agreeing to discuss it again at a future date helps to ensure that it will be acted on and is a well known way of improving time management. The co-tutoring process also models a lot of useful consulting skills. Indeed, a very similar process to co-tutoring has been used in Australia to help GP registrars learn consulting skills.[10]

The active listening process does not preclude challenge but the reason for the challenge is to facilitate the original speaker, not because the listener thinks he or she has a better idea. When it occurs it is often after careful reflection and thought on the part of the listener. It can help identify problems and allow the recognition of some strong feelings, and although our example was fictitious, it well illustrates this process.

DOES CO-TUTORING WORK?

There are a number of components to the co-tutoring process – active listening, reflection, summarizing, support, time and task management, feedback, challenge and action planning. The effect of these in bringing about creative change is hard to assess directly. We have reports of participants dealing with various personal crises, illness, changing practices, planning career development, undertaking postgraduate degrees and conducting audits and research. They claim that co-tutoring was important for them in dealing with these often very difficult issues. Some evidence for the success of co-tutoring comes from a survey carried out in our region in 1996.[11] Twenty-two out of 42 co-tutors reported that they were less stressed than before they started co-tutoring, with a further 18 reporting the same stress and only two feeling more stressed. This was at a time when stress in the profession was rising rapidly.

Why do we consider our approach to be so useful? The following are some observations about general practitioners and their professional development with which you might agree:

- GPs are often isolated despite working in partnerships. Relationships between partners are often less than ideal.
- GPs listen to a large number of patients every day. GPs are rarely listened to.
- Many GPs are stressed and most cope with it but few deal with it.
- GPs are practised at offering others support but find it hard to seek it themselves.
- Stressed GPs are least able to recognize their own problems and solve them.
- GPs tend to be very self-critical and dwell on negatives.
- GPs fear criticism from others often due to humiliating experiences during medical education.
- GPs find it hard to give and receive positive and, particularly, negative feedback constructively.
- GPs want to further their education but are often blocked by some of the above difficulties.

These factors inhibit growth and change in an individual's personal and professional life. Support and positive regard from colleagues can reverse this inhibition and empower doctors to realize their full potential, particularly as:

- Personal and professional development are inexorably linked especially in a discipline like general practice, which centres on interpersonal interaction.
- Individual adult learners need to discover solutions to their problems. They cannot have them externally imposed.[12] This discovery can be facilitated by active listening.
- General practice is not a hierarchical profession but assumes a parity between established practitioners. It requires a mode of continuing professional development that reflects that parity.
- GPs have enormous experience in helping people with problems. Unfortunately their ability fully to understand their patients can be

constrained by an emphasis on problem solving and other doctor-centred approaches.[13] In many instances active listening can be much more effective.

These are some of the ideas which led us to the concept of a support system that is entirely peer based and avoids what we see as the potentially hierarchical structure of mentor and mentee. This parity has a similarity to co-counselling and it has given rise to the name co-tutoring.

We feel that the mutual nature of the relationship is more than just paying lip service to the ethos of the profession, but that it confers some very tangible benefits. As the service is reciprocal, there is no need for payment to the mentor. This is an important consideration with regard to the long term financial feasibility of a mentoring scheme. More importantly, by denying the concept of an expert with the answers, co-tutoring encapsulates a relationship based on mutual listening and not finding solutions for the other person's problems. Here the theory of co-tutoring comes close to much of the later work of Carl Rogers, who saw the mutual offering of empathy, positive regard and congruence as a powerful vehicle for learning and change.[14]

TRAINING FOR CO-TUTORING

How can participants become proficient in co-tutoring? We think it is essential to start with a 2-day course, preferably residential. This gives participants time to:

- Gain an understanding of the co-tutoring process
- Acquire the basic skills necessary for it
- Decide if they wish to continue co-tutoring
- If so, decide with whom they might wish to work in a co-tutoring pair, trio or quartet.

The course is modelled throughout on the co-tutoring process and consists largely of exercises in pairs with one participant acting as speaker at any one time and the other as listener. A third participant may be present as an observer to help with feedback. In each exercise each participant has a chance to be speaker, listener and (where relevant) observer. We have found that two facilitators are essential in order to support each other and help to model the co-tutoring process.

After an introductory session to set the climate, the areas we try and include are listening and feedback skills, action planning, the effects of feelings and how self-disclosure can be made safe. The course ends with a session in which participants are helped to choose with whom they might wish to co-tutor. This choosing process can give rise to strong feelings which it is important to acknowledge and deal with. Sometimes the commitment to a co-tutoring relationship can seem daunting, and in order to minimize this understandable anxiety we suggest that the initial commitment is only until the group meets again for a follow-up day about 3 months later.

In practice most people have been keen to continue with their original co-tutoring partner(s) well beyond the first follow up day. They have also found it useful to continue meeting as a large group, with the original facilitators, about twice a year. These meetings help to foster supportive relationships within the wider group and allow for the development of co-tutoring skills.

ROLE OF FACILITATORS

As our experience with co-tutoring has grown, so has our realization that setting up and facilitating the scheme requires specific skills and experiences. Co-tutoring is primarily an experiential activity amongst peers. Therefore it is important that all facilitators should have had experience of working in this way. Co-tutoring requires openness and a preparedness to share vulnerability, so facilitators must be able to be honest about themselves and their own experience. Perhaps most crucially, the facilitators must have the ability to create and maintain safety for the participants without removing the challenge of pushing out the boundaries as to what is just comfortable. Inevitably, during workshops and working in small groups, participants may discover areas of distress and discomfort which can cause difficulties for themselves and others if they are frightened by, and inexperienced in, dealing with emotion. The facilitators need to be able to recognize what is going on for all participants, as well as themselves, and be able to handle it constructively. For this reason we believe that the facilitators should have had experience and training in counselling skills and have acquired a commitment to maintain a high degree of self knowledge.

These requirements are by no means restricted to doctors. The facilitation team is stronger for diversity. Most courses have two facilitators which we try and ensure comprise one doctor and one non-doctor as well as one of each sex. This can be particularly important in groups where the sex divide is unequal and participants are liable to feel isolated in issues that relate to gender.

We intend to research further the skills, knowledge and experience necessary for co-tutoring facilitation and to provide training to enable our experience to be shared with new facilitators.

EXPERIENCE OF CO-TUTORING

Co-tutoring has been going since 1994. Over 130 people have now been involved, some for over 3 years. As one of the central features of co-tutoring is that each individual has different needs, it is to be expected that experiences of co-tutoring will also vary. The practical arrangements of when, where and how frequently to meet are specific to the circumstances of those concerned. Some successful partnerships have conducted most of their contact through letters and phone calls, though the majority meet face to face perhaps once every 1–2 months. Some co-tutors also meet socially and a few have benefited from visiting each other's practices. These activities can be valuable but we feel that it is important to separate them from the actual co-tutoring sessions. At the outset the biggest hurdle can be the logistics of arranging meetings. As the relationships gel and the participants feel the benefits, the incentive to continue is maintained. Inevitably some partnerships never get off the ground due to incompatibility but this seems to have been less of a problem in the more recent courses where the process of choosing has been improved.

POTENTIAL DIFFICULTIES

Our experience as facilitators and that of many of the participants is that co-tutoring is a valuable process that can contribute significantly to the quality of professional practice with benefit for patients, practitioners and the service as a whole. What issues, then, still need to be considered?

Co-tutoring is not an easy option. It takes time, commitment and a certain amount of money, particularly in the first year when there are more workshops. GPs' time is already very heavily committed and those who would benefit from it the most may be those who find it the hardest to get away from their practices. Many are not used to paying the full cost of their education and go for the cheapest options, often with a preference for lecture formats rather than interactive learning.[15]

Concern has been expressed that co-mentoring schemes may lead to collusion and lack of rigour.[16] In addition to the essential separation of the speaker and listener roles, we believe that in our scheme there are three factors which can help to guard against this: firstly, the follow-up workshops where participants work with people other than their regular partners and are challenged as to the appropriateness of their co-tutoring; secondly, having a third person in a co-tutoring group helps give a broader perspective; finally, the facilitators are available to offer feedback on a couple's or trio's co-tutoring process (though we must admit that few groups have so far taken up this offer).

Some people have expressed concern that the process is too much like counselling and not education. Perhaps a useful way of regarding this issue is to think of the outcome of co-tutoring sessions. If, during the session, counselling skills have been used to facilitate a person's clear thinking and lead to a positive outcome, then well and good. The counselling skills can be regarded as just an extra tool for the listener. In fact, a common request from participants in later follow-up courses is to develop more counselling skills.

As facilitators we have debated this issue vigorously among ourselves. Indeed, three of us are experienced practitioners of co-counselling, on which much of co-tutoring is based. Yet the two who are not involved in co-counselling are equally convinced of the value of co-tutoring in furthering the professional and personal development of GPs. Whether such growth is as the result of 'counselling' or 'education' seems to us to be immaterial. What is important is that successful education requires a preparedness to change. Such change can appear threatening if the individual is feeling overwhelmed and stressed. Co-tutoring attempts to address these stresses and help people to change.

WHERE NEXT?

Where does co-tutoring fit into professional life? Our belief is that it is a learning process that is widely applicable both to GPs and other professionals. We would like it to become part of a constellation of peer supported learning schemes such as conventional mentoring. However it is also crucial that in the new world, where education will probably be linked to reaccreditation, any element of summative assessment is kept well clear of the co-tutoring relationship, as that would fundamentally distort the essence of it. As co-tutoring seems to be addressing the very problems that are causing the most anxiety to the profession, the patients and the government, it deserves the support of all three groups. While their concerns might be the same, their perspectives and assumptions will differ. The profession wants protected time and financial support to allow GPs to further their education. The government needs to improve the recruitment and retention of competent caring professionals but does not want to spend any extra money. As a culture we do not appear to trust the process of self-motivated adult learning and often rely on dictated wisdom. There will have to be negotiation and compromise between the various views to get the level of support and acceptance that is necessary. There is a need to develop a mode or modes of co-tutoring that can meet people where they are in terms of their educational perceptions and expectations. To do that we need to understand the process better and explore new ways of interpreting the theory to suit individual practice.

Acknowledgement

The members of the East Anglian Co-Tutoring Team who contributed this description of their work are Marion Barnett, Dr Andrew Easthaugh, Sue Parlby, Dr Paul Paxton and Dr Paul Sackin.

References

1 Hofstede G. 1991 *Cultures and Organizations*. McGraw-Hill International, UK
2 Ibid
3 Bond M.H. 1991 *Beyond the Chinese Face – Insights from Psychology*. Oxford University Press, Oxford
4 Personal discussion 14. 8. 97 (Newham)
5 Pugh D.S. and Hickson D.J. 1989 *Writers on Organizations*, 4th edn. Penguin Business, UK
6 Ibid p. 119
7 Allen I. 1994 *Doctors and their Careers – A New Generation*. Policy Studies Institute, London
8 Conway C. 1994 *Mentoring Managers in Organizations*. Ashridge Printers, Berkhamstead
9 See for example Jain C., Narayan N., Narayan P. *et al.* 1985 Attitudes of Asian patients in Birmingham to general practitioner services. *Journal of Royal College of General Practice*, **35**, 416–18
10 Greco M, Buckley J. and Francis W. 1997 Triads – an effective method for learning the art of listening. *Education for General Practice*, **8**, 329–34
11 Hibble A. and Berrington R. 1998 Personal professional learning plans – an evaluation of mentoring and co-tutoring in General Practice. *Education for General Practice*, **9**, 216–21

12 Brookfield S. 1986 *Understanding and Facilitating Adult Learning*. Open University Press, Milton Keynes

13 Launer J. and Lindsey C. 1997 Training for systemic general practice: a new approach from the Tavistock Clinic. *British Journal of General Practice*, **47**, 453–6

14 Rogers C. 1980 *A Way of Being*. Houghton Mifflin, Boston MA

15 Murray T. and Campbell L. 1977 Finance not learning needs makes general practitioners attend courses – a data base survey. *British Medical Journal*, **315**, 353

16 1993 Report of a working group on higher professional education: *Portfolio Based Learning in General Practice*. Occasional Paper No. 63, Royal College of General Practitioners, London

9

A practical guide for mentor scheme leaders

Objectives

Holistic mentoring is designed as an intervention which makes a significant contribution to the wellbeing and professional development of individual practitioners, the recipients of mentoring. It is also designed to utilize the experience of becoming a mentor, to extend the mentor's own personal and professional development, so that both parties benefit from their mentoring relationship. Through this process, good mentor practice in an organization is established, and further dimensions of learning explored. This in turn feeds into the organization as a whole, offering new perspectives on responding to and resolving problems, making a further contribution towards positive outcomes of organizational change.

Step 1: Planning and preparation

For these spirals of experience, reflection, implementation, and evaluation to have an impact on an organization, they will have begun with planning and preparation time set aside to consider how these ultimate benefits can be achieved in your own particular work setting. You need to clarify what you want to achieve, and then how you are going to achieve it. Like reflection, setting time aside to get into this first spiral is often forfeited for the instant approach, the pitfalls of which have been described in the early chapters.

So, get into the first spiral by setting time aside, away from the workplace, to meet with other colleagues interested in mentoring, and over a few decent bottles of wine, consider some of these opening questions. Unless you devote a day to it, you won't get through them all in one go – a natural break occurs *after* point 4 (documentation).

Why now – what has prompted us to think seriously about introducing mentors?
What do we want mentoring to achieve?
Is mentoring the appropriate intervention to achieve this – or could it be achieved in some other way?
Where will the time come from?
Who would mentors be? Where and how would mentors be trained?
If we set up a mentor scheme – how would we evaluate it?

You might find it useful to refer to Jackie Bould's *Mentoring in Medicine* (listed in Essential reading section below), particularly pages 7–9.

Step 2: Planning analysis

To take your thinking further, try a SWOT analysis: brainstorm answers and ideas in these four areas:

Strengths: What will work for us in this endeavour?
Weaknesses: What will work against us?
Opportunities: Is there a window of opportunity open?
Threats: Are there factors/people likely to sabotage the initiative?

   At this point, it might be useful to summarize where you have got to, and bear in mind the following:

COMMON PROBLEMS FOUND IN PLANNED MENTORING PROGRAMMES[1]

1. The assumption that mentoring is obvious – anyone can do it
2. Insufficient numbers of qualified mentors
3. Inadequately prepared participants.

'in most instances it would be better not to implement a low-cost plan which neither adequately prepares participants (mentors) nor informs others about the intent and impact of their effort'[2]

and keep these thoughts in mind as you move into:

Step 3: Planning a structure

The previous analysis should have identified more clearly the resources available to you for your mentor scheme. There will never be sufficient, and if you wait until there are, you will never get started! Hopefully, reading this book will have helped your initial thinking about the constraints of your own work context, and how you might adapt to them without losing the distinctive features of the mentoring relationship.
   One of the messages of this book has been the importance of having a clear and manageable administrative structure to support your initiative, and this is more effectively accomplished when you have identified two major players: the project leader and the project co-ordinator.

The project leader

PERSON PROFILE

- A strong personal commitment to the vision of mentoring
- Prepared to go that extra mile when the occasion demands (it will)
- See the mentor scheme as a priority in their work
- Possess relevant knowledge and skills.

DISCUSSION POINT

Think laterally when sorting out who might be in line for this difficult but immensely rewarding task. Traditionally, practitioners who have educational roles in their region (GP tutors, trainers) are viewed as naturally the 'right' person for this type of group facilitation. In both mentor teams who have been the major protagonists in this book, leadership responsibility lies with practitioners who are simply established practitioners, and respected mentors. These practitioners have shown themselves to have the requisite skills in group work, coupled with the sort of clarity and insight which makes for very effective team working – they were just keeping quiet about it.

TASKS OF THE PROJECT LEADER

- Oversee the administrative structure of the project, delegating tasks appropriately
- Work closely with the identified project co-ordinator to keep an overview of the project's progress
- Set, and circulate dates for regular support meetings for mentors
- Devise the content and structure of mentor training programmes
- Facilitate the continuing learning-from-experience of the mentor team, identifying themes for further learning and development
- Be available to mentors in between formal meetings for advice and additional support
- Define and incorporate relevant evaluation procedures
- Disseminate the mentor project's experience to the profession.

TIME

Given the variations in the size of the mentor team, geographical location, already available administrative support, etc., it is difficult to be precise, but based on a team of 16 mentors working with 75 mentees, we would suggest four sessions per month as a reasonable starting point, assuming that goodwill provides for a reasonable overspill of time.

The project co-ordinator/administrator

PERSON PROFILE

- An interest in the concept of mentoring, and commitment to the project
- Sensitivity and warmth
- A sense of humour
- Can act on own initiative
- Can be reasonably flexible about working hours.

TASKS OF THE PROJECT CO-ORDINATOR/ADMINISTRATOR

- Writing to prospective new mentees and allocating to mentors
- Keeping the database of the project with detailed information on mentor/mentee pairings

- Preparing publicity material: flyers/posters/advertisements/newsletters
- Working with the project leader to arrange mentor team meetings, training meetings for new GP mentors, conferences, workshops
- PGEA for all meetings
- Attendance at team meetings
- Liaising with financial administrators if reimbursement is provided.

TIME

To make things considerably easier for potential project co-ordinators, we have developed a mentoring database. This centralized system has been designed to be very user friendly and significantly reduces the time needed to administer and co-ordinate the scheme to about 10 hours per week. Our database consultant is available to develop the existing frame-work for other mentoring schemes and details are included in the Appendices.

DISCUSSION POINT

Reference to the importance of this role is in Chapter 3 Part 1.

Allocating the administration of your project to an administrator who is already overworked risks losing the all-important, prompt follow-up of enquiries from potential mentees. This is an essential part of establishing your scheme, and advertising its credibility – mentees who fail to get a prompt response are quick to voice their frustration.

Step 4: Documentation

Examples of the documentation referred to in this book are placed in the appendices. These include:

Mentoring fact sheet – information sent to mentees
Interview recording sheet – used by both parties to record intentions, actions and working themes
Anonymous exit questionnaire – sent to the mentee when the mentoring work is concluded, to enquire about their experience of the scheme
Criteria for mentor team – a statement of accountability for a funding body
Database information
Questionnaire used by external evaluators.

Step 5: Defining the mentor role

Chapter 2 provides a sufficient overview of mentor roles, which alongside your previous analysis and discussion, should enable you to:

- Write a statement of the aims and objectives of the mentor's intervention

- Prepare written information to be given to potential mentees which includes:

  Ongoing nature of the relationship
  Confidential
  Voluntary
  Agenda set by mentee
  No feedback to 'authority'.

If your project is funded through the offices of the Dean of Postgraduate General Practice Education, or other institutional bodies, there may be a request for your project to fall into line with existing requirements for accountability. This means that you need to be ready to make overt and formal the criteria which you expect your mentor team to work to. An example of this sort of written criteria – in effect an agreement between the 'commissioners' and the 'providers' – is included in the 'examples of documentation' section in the appendices.

Step 6: Recruiting mentors and mentees

The more representative your mentor team in terms of professional age and stage, the richer and more varied the learning that is accrued, the more the profession will see mentoring as an internal support structure, to be undertaken by 'ordinary' established practitioners. With this in mind:

- How can you advertise beyond known sources?
- Are you going to include retired practitioners? If so, are there particular conditions, i.e. still in touch with practice through locum work?
- How 'experienced' must your mentors be – what about young practitioners?
- Do you need to consider targeting women deliberately, or practitioners from other cultures – if so, how?
- If you are able to offer some financial reimbursement to mentors, have you agreed the level and method of claiming it?
- How and when will you recruit your mentees?
- How will mentors be allocated to mentees?

Step 7: Selecting mentors

As previous chapters have shown, the effectiveness of the mentoring relationship relies less on the age, sex, and culture of origin of the mentor than on their possession of certain qualities that can translate into requisite skills. Summarizing the likely benefits of mentoring is a forerunner to considering the likely attributes of a mentor:

Benefits

FOR THE PERSON BEING MENTORED

Encourage reflection on practice
Identify areas for development
Provide a safe place for analysing current problems and concerns
Provide problem solving support, and information
Career guidance and advice
Develop insight and strategies in problem solving
Assist and support the change process
Encourage self confidence and ownership of the future.

FOR THE MENTOR

Enhance job satisfaction
Develop interpersonal skills
Encourage self-reflection and reflection on own practice
Develop problem-solving abilities
Encourage own further professional development
Further a sense of collegiality through shared tasks
Develop self confidence
Expansion of work roles.

Attributes

Likely attributes found in a mentor become more transparent when you consider the outcomes that you are working towards. Some of the 'hard' areas – like career guidance, or identifying areas for development, can be seen as information-giving, requiring an informed, up-to-date practitioner, but these have to be balanced with attributes that take the mentor into 'soft' areas like analysing current concerns, or reflection on practice, requiring sensitivity and personal warmth.

But, given that the experience of mentoring in itself shift attitudes, and changes perspectives, and providing you intend to put in place the requisite structures for supporting and developing mentors, you can extend your selection of mentors to include those who demonstrate their *potential* for developing the following attributes, as well as those who come 'ready-made', as it were. From experience, we would offer these attributes as being desirable in a mentor:

- Team players – meaning that they enjoy being part of a team, and are prepared to compromise their individual wants to the collective good
- Prepared to be open themselves, willing to share their experience, and learn from their peers
- Flexible in their thinking, open to alternative explanation
- Have a commitment to supported learning and development
- Have the respect of their peers
- Good communicators, sensitive to their own conduct with others
- Share in the vision of mentoring as a tool for professional development
- Prepared to give time and energy to the task.

Disabling mentors

By the same token, it becomes transparent that some attitudes are undesirable in mentors, leading to the 'toxic' mentors referred to by Neil Munro in Chapter 6. These include:

- Concrete thinkers – those with rigid, inflexible thinking patterns, wedded to the rightness of their own view and unable to hear and consider alternative views
- Power seekers – using the mentor role as a means of enhancing personal power and control in the organization
- Controllers – using the mentoring relationship as a directive means to enforcing their own agenda
- Poor communicators – those who remain inaccessible to others.

Now you have got your group of mentors, hopefully clear about their role, and enthused with the concept of mentoring. The final step in this do-it-yourself guide is to offer a suggested framework for an induction workshop for your identified mentors.

Induction workshop for mentors

Having identified your mentor team, it is useful to set aside a day for an induction workshop. This workshop can both help establish the group, providing an opportunity to begin to develop a collective identity, as well as clarify the task and the requisite skills. It ensures that everyone starts from the same place, as it were.

For those unsure about where to start, the following text offers a framework for an induction workshop, including some relevant exercises. For those who simply want to take on the task of becoming a mentor without reference to others, then reading through the framework should promote some more thinking about your skills and identity as a mentor.

Suggested framework

This workshop is based on a 1-day event lasting 6–7 hours. The ideal group size for this type of event is 12 or less; more than that, and it becomes difficult to manage an effective overview of the process. If your resources run to it, it is well worth considering an overnight stay, which provides a better quality of protected time to develop discussion and experience, and is invaluable in consolidating the team. You will need two rooms (for small group work), or at the very least a room large enough for participants to work privately, in corners, or make use of corridors or other informal space.

TASK 1: INTRODUCTIONS

An opening exercise which gives everyone a chance to introduce themselves and share something about their life with each other is an important feature of creating a learning climate of trust and support. GP Course

Organizers are a good resource if you are stuck for an opening exercise; otherwise you can try this one:

Ask participants to pair off, getting them to work with an unknown person where possible. Be steadfast in the face of any initial reluctance to leave the safety of their chairs, and the handbook which you have so thoughtfully provided, encouraging participants to abandon both, and find a partner. When they are paired off, and settled into a quiet space with their partner, set the task. It is worth writing it up on a flip chart, so that participants can refer to it as they move through the various stages.

1. Tell the participants that at the end of this exercise you will be asking them to introduce their partner to the rest of the group, and say something about them. Say that you will keep the time boundaries (easier to do if you do not yourself join in on the exercise, but feed in information about yourself at the end of the group round).
2. Talk to your partner. Apart from the usual professional stuff about where they trained, where their practice is, etc. find out:

   Their name – the name that they want us to use in this workshop
   Something interesting about them; an interesting aspect of themselves which they are prepared for the group to know about
   Why they came to this workshop.

3. After 15 minutes call time, and make sure they change over, so that the other partner now has a chance to talk about themselves.

Time for this phase: 30 minutes

4. Now ask each participant to introduce their partner to the group. Note preference for names, and scribe up headlines of why they came to the workshop, so that you and they can check their initial motivation with their learning as the day unfolds. Time for this phase depends on the personalities of your participants; usually each pair takes on average 5 minutes.

Time for this phase: 60 minutes. A coffee break here fits nicely

TASK 2: QUALITIES AND DEFINITIONS OF A MENTOR

Once the ice is broken, you can get into the business of forming a collective view of a mentor. You can build on the previous exercise in this way:

1. Have a round of names to help fix them in participants' minds. After this, pair off the pairs – making three small groups of four. Ask each small group to appoint a scribe; someone who will present the themes of their discussion at the end of the exercise.
2. Through shared discussion, the task for the small groups is to:

   • Identify a person (or people) who have acted as mentors, either formally or informally, at any stage of their life. Ask participants to describe these mentors to their peers in the small group.

- What did these mentors offer? What qualities did they possess? What was it about them that makes them stand out?

3. Ask each group to make a list of the mentor qualities that were identified through discussion.

Time for this phase: 30 minutes

4. Ask each group to present their list of qualities, pausing for discussion and clarification as they are presented.
5. Use the collated list of qualities to begin a brainstorm – a spontaneous discussion on the participants' definition of a 'mentor'.

Finally, use their definitions to lay alongside your own. Introduce your definition of the task, and move into a description of the task of the mentor team within the context of your own work – in effect, introduce them to your mentor project.

Time for this phase: between 30 and 60 minutes

TASK 3: REQUISITE SKILLS

Previous discussion should have elicited whether you have a (more or less) collective definition of the mentor's role, enabling you to assess how far (or otherwise) you as leader and your team are in step. You should also have a fair spread of mentor attributes, which frequently overlap into skills. Once you are confident that you are all talking about the same thing, you are in a good position to move into considering requisite skills.

It is beyond the scope of this chapter to offer a distance learning module on communication skills. The books listed as essential references all include good descriptions of communication skills necessary for mentors, and these can be compared with the profession's own knowledge and experience of teaching communication skills to registrars on vocational training schemes.

Chapter 3 gives descriptions of requisite skills, and a three-stage model for developing them. But, to emphasize the importance of sensitive communication to potential mentors, it's worth considering drawing their attention to the importance of attentive, empathic listening, not least because doctors are most frequently in the role of prescribing 'tellers'. Listening without distortion, giving space and encouragement to a speaker to unfold their tale, and refraining from interrupting them whilst they do so are first level skills, but pretty difficult to achieve. You can demonstrate this in a number of ways, but the following exercise is useful to lay the foundation:

The 'tape recorder' exercise
Inform participants of the objective of the exercise, which is to rehearse listening without distortion, test accurate recall, and provide a summarized review of what has been heard. Again, you need to stay outside and manage the exercise, and the time boundaries.

Put your participants into trios, and ask them to label themselves as A, B, and C:

A is the tape recorder
B is the teller
C is the non-participant observer.

For 5 minutes, B tells A what motivated them to become a general practitioner.

A listens without interruption, offering non-verbal encouragement only.

If the teller finishes telling before the 5 minutes is up, ask them to sit quietly and reflect on what they have been saying. However, it is worth strongly encouraging people to continue to use the time – even if initially they feel they have no more to say. This encourages development, and reflection on themes.

At the end of 5 minutes *A acts as a tape recorder*. He/she feeds back to their partner what they have heard, recounting as much as they can recall. When they have finished feeding back, they hold up their hand.

When their hand is raised, *the observer* moves in. The observer's task is to:

1. Check for distortion – did the tape recorder play back what was actually said, or what the receiver (tape recorder) heard?
2. Fill in any missing part of the story.

No more than 3 minutes for this – try to make sure observers keep to this task, and don't deviate into their own agenda about how it all came about, etc. There is time for this later.

When the observer has given feedback, they ask *B – the teller* – 'how did it feel to hear your story played back?'

Again, no more than 3 minutes – ask both the tape recorder and the observer to simply listen without comment to this feedback.

Repeat the exercise until all three participants have had the experience of being teller, tape recorder, and observer.

Time for this part of the exercise (allowing for 15 minute cycles) 45 minutes

You now start to take feedback from each trio about:

What did it feel like to be the teller – to have uninterrupted time to tell a story?
What sort of non-verbal cues did they search for in their listener?
Did they recognize their story when it was played back to them – did it sound different in any way?
What it was like to be the tape recorder:

Did anxiety about remembering cloud their initial listening?
How did they select what they retained?
Did anyone write down notes – if so what effect did it have on the
teller?

Points to make following discussion:

Distortion: 'a man hears what he wants to hear and disregards the rest'
The importance of accurate listening, and feedback – voice inflections
which alter meanings: 'this is what I heard – is this what you said?'
Selective attention – what we remember, and why
Attention – listening at this level is exhausting
Non-verbal cues that are encouraging to the teller – and identify some of
those that are unhelpful and hinder the process.

Time allowed for feedback phase: 30 minutes

TASK 4: REHEARSING THE MENTOR ROLE – THE REFLECTIVE CYCLE

The previous exercise, or one of the many others that have a similar aim, is
a good lead into trying out the Reflective Cycle as a means of getting into
the mentoring position. But the ground rules for using it have to be clearly
established:

- Introduce the Reflective Cycle, and say something about its conceptual
  base to put it into context for participants, most of whom will not have
  read the book! Circulate participants with copies of the Reflective Cycle,
  and the specimen open-ended questions attached.
- Put participants into pairs – leave the choice of a partner to them. They
  might wish to return to their partner of the introductory phase, or want
  to work with someone new.

Explain that, as time does not allow for more than one area of the Cycle
to be explored, each person will decide on *one* area to work in with their
partner. Their partner will take on the role of mentor, exploring their
chosen area with them, using the open-ended questions supplied, or
devising their own.

- Half an hour is allocated to each person for this work. After half an hour
  of exploration, there will be 5 minutes for both recipient and mentor to
  reflect on their experience. After reflection, the pairs change roles, so
  that the person who acted as 'mentor' to their partner now becomes
  the recipient, choosing their area of work in the same way as before,
  so that at the end of the rehearsal exercise, each participant has had
  the experience of acting as mentor, asking open-ended questions
  and exploring life events, and being on the receiving end of reflective
  exploration.
- Make clear that as the group leader, or facilitator, you do not intend to
  enquire into the *content* of the rehearsal, but would like feedback on
  the *experience* of using the Cycle. You can use this as a demonstration
  of how mentoring experience can be shared, without invading the privacy, and confidentiality of the relationship. However, some participants

will be quite happy to share the content, at least in part, to illustrate their experience of using the Reflective Cycle, and if they do so, make sure that the group honours this as shared learning.

- Finally, to confirm the privacy of the exercise, explain that you intend to keep out of their way, and not eavesdrop in their agenda. You will monitor time boundaries, and ensure that they have a place in which they can work quietly and without interruption.

Time for this phase: minimum 75 minutes, ideally 90 minutes to allow for slippage

- Feedback phase. You will probably have been frantically rounding up the pairs in the meantime, but it is important to make sure the group has time to come back together, and share the experience. You can do this fairly informally, by asking participants:

- What did their mentor do that was helpful to the process of telling their story?
- What did their mentor do that was less helpful, and hindered their telling?
- How would they describe the experience of being listened to?
- How was the sequence of open-ended questions managed?

Time for this phase: 20–30 minutes

TASK 5: REVIEWING THE EXPERIENCE OF THE WORKSHOP, AND LOOKING AHEAD

It is important to leave time to close the workshop carefully, reviewing the learning and experience of the day, and building a bridge into your implementation of the scheme. Make sure that you:

- Summarize the main themes of the day for participants
- Ask participants to evaluate the day (you can use a written format for this, or seek verbal feedback)
- Stress again that the workshop was intended as a taster – participants can opt out of becoming a mentor if they feel it is not for them
- Explain the procedure for those who do wish to continue and become mentors in your project.

  Draw their attention to the date of the first mentor meeting, and explain that this is purposefully timed to take place soon after they have conducted their first mentoring interview. Remember that a time lapse of longer than 2 months between your induction workshop and the first mentor team meeting will jeopardize the enthusiasm and energy for the task which your induction workshop has produced
- Allow time for questions and clarification of earlier points.

Time for this final phase: minimum 30 minutes

If one of the main objectives of this book has been met, then mentor project leaders will have gleaned some information which prompts their thinking on how to do and not to do things. As for what follows after in

your mentoring scheme, we can offer no practical guide, only encouragement to realize the shared benefits of mentoring by reaching beyond the
obvious, and with a near aim explore the main chance of things as yet
not come to life.

Essential reading

Apart from Shakespeare, who undoubtedly knew a lot about mentoring,
the following books offer help and ideas about the process of mentoring,
and the requisite skills, and are useful reading for mentor scheme leaders
and the mentor team:

1. Although from a nursing background, Anne Palmer and Alison
   Morton-Cooper's *Mentoring and Preceptorship*, published by Blackwell
   Science, is well structured and informed, with an excellent and well-
   ordered bibliography for further reading. There are useful chapters on
   the learning environment, and a chapter which sets out useful distinctions between the various support roles.
2. *Mentoring in Medicine: a Practical Guide* written by Jackie Bould, and
   published through the CCDU Training and Consultancy based at the
   University of Leeds. This is a very practical guide, aimed at hospital
   staff, which sees the mentor's role as one which includes appraisal
   but it provides useful examples of mentor contracts and agreements,
   and the practical, step-by-step layout of the book encourages a professional, well-structured model of intervention.
3. *Counselling Skills for Health Professionals*, written by Philip Burnard and
   published by Chapman and Hall, London, is a clear, easily accessible
   book which, as well as describing skills relevant to effective mentoring,
   raises (and answers) some interesting questions (for example, can you
   mentor a personal friend?), which new mentors particularly would
   find useful.
4. Finally, Gerard Egan's classic *The Skilled Helper – a Problem-Management
   Approach to Helping*, published by Brooks/Cole Publishing Company,
   California. This book addresses helping skills in greater depth and
   breadth, for example setting out the process of effective challenging,
   and action planning and goal setting. In addition, there is some
   thought-provoking text on the ethics of helping, and the 'shadow
   side' of helping activity.

References

1 Phillips-Jones L. 1989 Common problems in planned mentoring programmes. *Mentoring
   International*, **3**(1), 36–40
2 Zey M.G. 1989 Building a successful formal mentor programme. *Mentoring International*,
   3(1), 48–51

___10___

Mentoring for professional development: Future visions and future threats

'There is a history in all men's lives
Figuring the nature of the times deceased
The which observed, a man may prophesy
With a near aim, of the main chance of things
As yet not come to life, which in their seeds
And weak beginnings lie intreasured.'

(Shakespeare *Henry IV* part 2)

Transformative power of mentoring

Now we are at the end – or, more properly, at another beginning – of our story.

At one level, this book has described the application of a style of intervention designed to maximize the potential benefits that mentoring can bring to both parties in the relationship. Underpinning this is a belief, supported by findings from other professions as well as our own experience, that, when properly conducted, mentoring is a worthwhile activity. At another level, the story has told the tale of a group of people who set out on a journey to build bridges, from which they learnt many things, and along the way discovered themselves.

Reflecting on the moral of the story highlights the components of the tale which are carried forward to become embodied in the story which still lies ahead, waiting to be told. Our first reflection is on the power of mentoring. It comes as no surprise to hear that doctors, like many before them, experience the 'feel good factor' produced by the catharsis of airing their current agenda with an attentive and encouraging listener. Indeed, judging by the mass of literature to this effect, we could confidently predict this to be an inevitable, as well as a desirable, outcome of a supportive discussion. We have seen, however, that holistic mentoring holds the capacity to realize far more than this. An effective mentoring relationship can engender in both mentor and mentee a greater vision of what they can accomplish professionally. This achieves the primary objective of 'professional development' – to find the 'possible self'. Possible selves[1] represent the individuals' ideas of what they might become, what they would like to become, and what they are afraid of becoming. Possible selves are important because they provide an evaluative and interpretive context for the current view of self, and function as incentives for future behaviour. The interaction of the mentoring relationship offers the opportunity for professional life to be reviewed, and significant life events revisited, making more visible the current view of self. From this quest come new insights, discoveries which provide new information with which to organize a life which can achieve a more comfortable fit between self and the outside world, and accommodate change.

In this opening exploration, a closer view of the possible future self is afforded. Standing alongside the view is the mentor, who makes an offer to act as guide in making the transition from current to future self. Not everyone will take up the offer, for some will prefer, for the time being at least, to stay where they are.

This accompanied transitional journey contains the transforming power of mentoring. The nature of the power is difficult to capture for description and measurement, yet it remains as a cardinal ingredient in distinguishing mentoring from other forms of helping intervention, and in achieving the transition from feeling good to being better. Whilst we can with great confidence assert that all 130 mentees using the scheme feel better for their mentoring relationship – less isolated, better able to manage stress, etc. – a more important claim is that a significant number of those mentees developed greater autonomy, the ability to act separately from the demands of their environment, and to move towards realizing their future selves. From this perspective, we could assume that they are better equipped to carry out the task of caring for patients with increased energy and confidence.

Transitional journeys

In a paper presented to the International Conference on Mentoring in April 1997, Professor Tony Dixon, speaking about his experience of training mentors to work within his Department of General Practice in Hong Kong University, saw transformation as a key concept in mentoring, and the journey as metaphor. He concluded that the distance between mentors and mentees was a critical factor in the transforming process. If the mentors had not themselves journeyed, made some paradigm shifts in their own understanding and knowledge, then 'the crucible was too cool – there is no light without heat'. The inference here is that without the mentor's own experience of transformation, they are less able to offer to their mentee that additional dimension which distinguishes mentoring from other forms of intervention, and makes it an immensely powerful tool for professional development. It is on this basis that we seek first of all to recruit new mentors from amongst those who have themselves received it – the mentees.

From this, we can see that it is insufficient to simply offer uncritical support to mentors as they pursue their task. Although, like cathartic listening, it promotes a 'feel good factor' and is certainly better than nothing at all, it cannot maximize the secondary benefit of mentoring, namely the professional development of the mentor, which in turn ensures that their mentee is sufficiently challenged by the heat and light of the crucible. Jung summarizes the challenge succinctly:

'We have learned to place in the foreground the personality of the doctor himself as the curative or harmful factor – what is now demanded is his [sic] own transformation the self-education of the educator'[2]

This story of mentoring gave some pictures of a continuous thread of initial training, support and development for mentors, aimed at taking them beyond the basic requirement of supportive listening and well-placed advice to becoming facilitators in the fullest sense of the word. Like the mentoring task, the education of mentors in itself sought to be visionary, offering a range of opportunities for different perspectives to be explored, and accompanying learning experiences undertaken. Such learning offers the mentors a chance to embark upon their own transitional journey. This, together with our collective experience of the mentoring relationship, has moved us beyond perceiving future evaluations as primarily summative, centred on accumulating evidence which 'proves' the positive outcome of mentoring, to a recognition of the importance of formative evaluation by which to identify with more certainty the criteria by which the transformative power of mentoring can be fully realized.

Power and equality in the mentoring relationship

When the mentor has undergone his or her own journey, they gain an additional dimension, which their mentee can, if they so decide, harness as a means by which to embark upon their own. The wisdom of the mentor stems not from greater power or knowledge, but from their own 'self-transcendence' in which they are able to move beyond individualistic concerns to make links with more collective, or universal, issues.[3] It is in this way that mentors are 'different' from their mentees – and by virtue of occupying a different role in the relationship. The role of mentor is neither better nor 'higher' than that of mentee; it is simply different.

For such a solidly hierarchical profession, medicine yields a highly ambivalent attitude towards power, with an apparent inbuilt aversion to hierarchical relationships, and a concomitant obsession with peer relationships, as if these in themselves guarantee a uniformity of experience which cancels out power.

From the mentor scheme's continuing evaluation of the intervention comes no evidence to suggest that mentees are disabled or disgruntled by matters of inequality. This may be due in part to the mentor's position of neutrality; they have no designated authority within existing hierarchical structures, and represent 'ordinary' but respected and credible general practitioners. Another likely reason is the independence of both sides. Equality in mentoring relationships lies not only in the shared power that brings benefits in learning to both partners, but also in the mentor's continual granting of autonomy to the recipient of their giving – the mentee. This is transferred through the mentor's consistent relinquishment of their own needs in order to focus on the mentee's agenda, secure in the knowledge that they can take their own agenda elsewhere. The mentor support group functions to offer the same scrutiny and support to the mentor as they offer to their mentee. Independence is furthered by the deliberate placing of the support system well outside the mentoring relationship, to avoid the collusive element commonly encountered in co-working, and frequently cited as a potentially limiting factor in self-development.

Visions and threats – relationship of mentoring to accountability

Whilst we have shown that this impartiality, and the absence of controlling power, is highly valued by mentees, we have discovered unforeseen obstacles to achieving it. The small size of some geographical areas will make it difficult to ensure the neutrality of the mentor, particularly in rural communities where the professional group is prominent, and its personalities well known. To fully realize the effectiveness of the mentoring relationship requires access to private worlds, and this is less likely to be granted when the mentor is perceived as someone whose previous and continuing knowledge of the mentee leads to preformed opinions and prejudiced perceptions. This risks mentoring being taken up as an extension of a social relationship, lacking the cutting edge of confrontation and challenge, and settling instead for a comfortable and collusive partnership.

We have also learnt that culture influences perceptions of power and authority, which, for mentors, requires of them another layer of necessary flexibility and understanding. The nature of authority becomes critical when considering the future role of a mentor in the process of professional accountability, currently part of the professional debate on the re-accreditation of practitioners.

There are differing views in the mentor teams regarding involvement in any future organizational system of professional accountability. Overall, mentors are relatively comfortable with the role of a mentor in developing the concept of portfolio learning, where their mentee might wish to include in the evidence of their continuing professional development a commentary on the learning outcomes of their mentoring relationship. This appears as a perfectly proper use of mentoring time, and a further realizable value of mentoring. Mentors are adamant, however, that if mentors became associated with a policing role, using the mentoring relationship to monitor competence, and importing into it an appraisal function, then this would destroy the voluntary, confidential, supportive nature of the mentoring alliance, thereby rendering the relationship invalid as a tool for professional development, and striking a death-blow to its future expansion.

Poorly performing doctors

For many mentors, it seems simpler to stand totally outside any activity whose primary goal is to gather evidence of continuing clinical competence, and evidence of continued learning and development. And yet, as this book goes to press, discussions with colleagues in the local medical committees and in health authorities are underway to address the possible future role of mentors in helping and supporting poorly performing doctors. As some mentors in the team begin to undertake this work, they are absolutely certain that the word 'mentor' must not be allowed to become associated with under-performance and disciplinary procedures. Mentoring is first and foremost an activity synonymous with voluntary, self-directed action, undertaken by functioning doctors intent on pursuing their own professional development, and promoting their present strengths. Whilst similar skills to those possessed by mentors can be usefully employed to support those who are known to be struggling to survive the demands of general practice, or those who are emerging from the trauma of disciplinary procedures, there needs to be a clear distinction between the two interventions. This could be achieved first and foremost by affording to those who offer such support a different title from that of mentor, for example that of professional supervisor, and secondly by ensuring that their job description describes and requires the different nature of their task.

The uneasiness of mentor practitioners about any future role in systems of accountability highlights the conflicting values of the right to privacy and the right to know. Readers will recall that this tension initially dogged the support groups, where the mentee's right to privacy was balanced against the need of the mentor to know how he or she was doing. Although doctors are familiar with receiving the personal disclosure of patients, information gathered as a mentor carries the status of private knowledge, and the obligation not to report it applies as much, if not more, inside the professional community as outside of it. Thus the report-back function of any appraisal sits uneasily with the equal, voluntary nature of the mentoring partnership.

Transforming a professional culture

These discussions serve to focus minds on the future capacity of mentoring as a preventive measure – which is, of course, where our story began, when the divisions made by the Devil's fingers became ravines, not just cracks in the profession's surface. And when Allah sent angels to help men and make things easier for them, so that they could cross the abyss, he cleverly realized that by doing so men would learn very quickly how to make things better for themselves, and that in time they could, if they worked hard, transform the whole land transversed by rivers and ravines, and bring about a transformation in the professional culture.

The implementation of the 1995 (Medical Performance) Act in September 1997 might go some way towards persuading funding bodies that the benefits obtained from a well-structured mentor scheme in terms of the retention and expansion of an empowered workforce far exceed the relatively small outlay of financing it. But implicit in the mentor's potential future as a form of insurance to prevent an undetected, but inexorable slide into professional chaos, is the challenge of educating the professional population to take up and use available mentoring programmes. Unfortunately, the legacy of professional training is such that doctors are unused to learning in depth, consistently, over time. They are more familiar with superficial learning styles, which maintain the divide between thinking and feeling, and keep the learner invisible. When something different is indicated, it naturally arouses uncertainty – every doctor should have a mentor, but what should they use them for?

The previous learning experience of most general practitioners will not have set the scene for the reflective exploration that precedes the transformative learning encountered in an effective mentoring relationship. Nor can we predict for a potential mentee what will come out of their mentoring, although now, at least, we can start to tell them what has come out of it for others, and how these outcomes were achieved. Perhaps some of those who read this story will feel encouraged to enter into the different experience of a mentoring journey, to trust in their own, and their mentor's capacity to realize a different sort of value. But the very essence of the mentoring relationship means that the proof of the pudding can only be found in the eating of it yourself.

It is in this broader sense that mentoring holds also the capacity to transform the organizational culture of general practice. We have seen that, when the window of opportunity was open in the crisis of change, mentors were sitting there – as Zen predicted, when the pupil is ready the lesson appears. Our experience strongly suggests that the organization is ready, and the lesson is underway. Mentors have addressed the individual factors that act as hindering forces, impeding professional development and change but, as the mentee in our story said, this is like a stone dropped into a pond; the collective action of mentoring will be the ripples which spread outwards, washing on to the wider shores of the organization. The mentor teams saw this possibility for themselves, as we heard early on in the story when they glimpsed a view of their future selves as change agents, bringing a more positive, warmer climate to general practice, and improving the likelihood of a higher outcome level following the crisis of imposed change.

The ripples are made more powerful when the activity is placed within the public domain of the professional community. Simons[4] believes that the transformation of professional values is widened by the activity of practitioner-led research and, when this is in progress, calls for a 'corresponding degree of insulation' from the technocratic systems of external surveillance and control currently evolving within the UK in response to accountability pressures. There is a parallel here between general practice, presently working towards establishing its own framework of accountability to avoid external surveillance and control, and MacDonald's[5] idea of schools as self-critical communities within high walls – groups who risk enough in collective self reflection to be spared the added risk of continuous exposure to outside observation. Holistic mentoring appears as a means of introducing into the profession a wider practice of reflection-on-action as a practitioner and as a person, thus uniting the professional and personal divide. By this means comes a possibility of dismantling a value structure based on privacy, territory, and hierarchy and replacing it with one which values openness and shared critical responsibility.

A further aspect of transforming the professional culture comes from the power of mentoring to re-import professional collegiality, through restoring the 'spirit of community'.[6] This is based on reciprocity, a sense of responsibility for the wellbeing of others, and an awareness that no-one is unaffected by the fate of others. In part, this comes from the open, shared, critical reflection of the holistic mentoring relationship, in part from the compassionate fellow feeling[7] intrinsic to the mentoring relationship. Pickering[8] himself shows this quality in his articulate plea to reinstate the word 'kindness' both in medical practice and in the professional journals, because its absence by name there, and in medical skills courses or other official edicts, implies that it is somehow unscientific; unworthy of the doctor's attention. Yet the author concludes that it 'is a supreme medical ally'. This story has shown that it is an equally powerful ally when applied to the practitioners themselves. A professional culture which encourages the display of kindness towards, and compassion between, its practitioners creates an ethos of mutual care and support. It restores consistency between the professional values of general practice, and the core values of the self, and from this comes the opportunity to represent human values in continuing medical education. Over time, these will be assimilated by the GP registrar, not through their intellectual faculty, but by the adaptation they make to the prevalent professional culture. Through the process of their own learning, their identification with, and their modelling on, the trainer/mentor as they make the transitional journey from journeyman/registrar to master/principal, similar values are carried forward into their own career.

New horizons

More pragmatically, and somewhat paradoxically to the sentiments which uphold the validity of insider-research, if mentoring is to have a stake in the future general practice community, it must be seen to respond to the continuing call for external accountability through the channels of funded research projects. These areas incorporate the observations of the external researchers writing in Chapter 7, and include:

- Identifying the long-term outcomes of mentoring
- Mentoring as a strategy for organizational development
- Comparing those GPs who take up mentoring with those who choose not to
- Issues of culture and gender in the mentoring relationship
- The impact of mentoring on structures for professional accountability
- A large scale evaluation of the impact of mentor schemes across the profession
- The kind of methods for research on mentoring which will advance current knowledge and debate.

Perversely, it is the very expansion of mentoring which overshadows its future – that together with confused terminology. Mentoring faces the danger of being perceived as a panacea for all ills, and therefore hastily applied – 'fervour without infrastructure'.[9] This leads to a further danger, namely that underfunded projects using untrained mentors with no thought of evaluation will reduce mentoring to a narrow, mechanized process which fulfils none of the unique opportunities described in our story. So mentoring comes with a health warning – unless it is properly resourced, delivered, administered and evaluated there will be significant problems in applying it as a resource for future needs.

Problems of future application are exacerbated by differing perceptions of what mentoring is, with an accompanying confusion in terminology, and this poses a threat to the useful outcome of any further research. The word 'mentor' is used to describe a myriad of activities, and looks set to share a similar fate to that of the word 'counsellor'. Both are words used as umbrella terms to embrace uncertain, ill-defined, or still-evolving activities. But, as the early studies which preceded this mentor scheme revealed, we are not all talking about the same thing. Then, and now, mentoring was not infrequently perceived and used as a one-off intervention to provide educational supervision, or as an ad hoc form of co-counselling. Unless there is some collective agreement to uphold the distinguishing features of mentoring which have been identified in this story – that it is a developing, continuing relationship which addresses the three components of education, development, and support necessary for professional growth, is non-hierarchical, neutral, objective; a relationship voluntarily entered into and focused on the needs of the mentee – then we have no common language from which to debate the issues. The concept of mentoring is eroded, and becomes diffuse, so that we are prevented from entering into the very discourse that will bring about its theoretical and practical expansion.

This is not just an academic debate, for a critical malfunction of such confusion is that it disables doctors from making accurate choices about the type of support they seek when facing the challenges of the next decade, and it becomes more vital as new ventures appear on the horizon. The holistic model of mentoring is being adopted and used by consultants and registrars in four of our hospital trusts, to support the development of junior doctors, and themselves. A further pilot project will look at the advantages or otherwise of using GP mentors, familiar with but outside the hospital context, to work as externally placed, objective mentors with junior hospital doctors.

The end of the beginning

Finally, having reflected on some of the underlying messages of the story, we must place it in a wider context by asking the questions:

What is the problem to which mentoring will be seen as the answer in the future?

Will mentors become gentle disciples of accountability, the velvet glove on the iron fist of reaccreditation?

Is the mentoring relationship in itself a means by which the troops are restrained from deserting their post, kept happy and quiescent by the mentor's tender loving care, a field dressing before being dispatched back to the front line?

Does mentoring serve as a device which maintains the professional status quo, preventing the sort of radical revolution which would overthrow the present orthodoxy of general practice and replace it with something other?

We hope that telling our story has served to strengthen a vision of mentoring as having the capacity to lay planks across the mountain streams and unite practitioners across their personal and professional divisions, so that they do not shout, or look in vain, but can cross more easily. In the future, providing that guardian angels care and maintain it, mentoring could become like the great construction of Mehmed Pasha, whose bridge still stands today, spanning the River Bosphorus in the glorious city of Istanbul.

Handicapped by having no personal knowledge of angels, it is difficult to judge if the mentors with whom I work are angelic. I suspect they are far too pragmatic, too involved in the real world, to earn that title. But if, as in the Arabic legend, angels are those who spread their wings over a divide, and teach men and women how to become bridge builders, then they are most certainly Arabic angels.

Myth is not limited by history but represents timeless truths. Those who build bridges bring manifold and unforeseen blessings to many people, no less than when they do so within a beleaguered profession. Rather than commit the sin of interference, we should resolve to keep building, and maintain the bridges made by mentors for as long as the profession ordains they should stand – as their predecessors did, in the name of Allah, the most compassionate, the most merciful.

References

1 Markus H. and Nurius P. 1986 Possible selves. *American Psychologist*, **41**(9), 954–969
2 Jung C. quoted in Sedgwick D. 1994 *The Wounded Healer – Countertransference from a Jungian Perspective*. Routledge, London, p. 7
3 Orwoll L. and Perlmutter M. 1990 The study of wise persons. In *Wisdom: its Nature, Origins and Development*. Cambridge University Press
4 Simons H. 1978 *Process Evaluation in Practice*. Mimeo Department of Curriculum Studies, University of London
5 MacDonald B. 1970 The evaluation of the Humanities Curriculum Project: a holistic approach. In *Theory into Practice*, Norwich CARE OCC Publ., University of East Anglia, Norwich
6 Etzioni A. 1993 *The Spirit Of Community: Rights, Responsibilities And The Communitarian Agenda*. Crown Publishers, New York
7 Taylor B 1997 Compassion: its neglect and importance. *British Journal of General Practice*, **47**, 521–3
8 Pickering W.G. 1997 Kindness, prescribed and natural, in medicine. *Journal of Medical Ethics*, **23**, 116–18
9 Gay B. 1997 The practice of mentoring. In *Mentoring – The New Panacea?* (ed. Stephenson J). Peter Francis Publishers

Appendix 1: Mentoring fact sheet

Why be a mentee?

Mentoring has been used as a means of supporting and developing staff in higher education for some time. There is increasing interest in the value of this activity for general practice, particularly at a time of change and stress in the profession as a whole. There are many potential benefits:

1. Mentees appreciate receiving the undivided attention of a fellow professional, who, whilst not a member of their practice, understands the complexities of their job, without being closely involved with particular agendas.
2. Mentees find mentoring sessions facilitate their professional development, help clarify educational needs, and offer a measure of personal support for them in their work.
3. Mentors find the experience of mentoring rewarding; it challenges and extends their own professional development. Mentees frequently use their own experience of being mentored to go on and become mentors themselves.

What is a mentor?

A mentor is an established practitioner, and respected peer, who offers, through an ongoing professional relationship with his or her mentee, opportunities to develop, stimulate and maintain their professional development by:

- Discussing any current professional concerns
- Providing space and time to reflect on, and evaluate their work
- Helping to identify further learning needs
- Offering help and support with personal and professional development.

All mentors in the South Thames (West) mentor team are trained, and supported in their work by the Educational Adviser, herself an experienced mentor.

Where and when does mentoring take place?

The decision as to how often you meet with your mentor is for you both to decide, based on your individual requirements. Generally, mentoring meetings take place about four or five times a year. The meetings usually need at least an hour and a half. The meeting place is a mutually convenient one – although your mentor might suggest a 'neutral' meeting place, away from the hassles of the workplace. As mentoring sessions are considered a professional activity, social venues are usually avoided.

How does mentoring work?

As the mentee, you decide the content and agenda of your session – your mentor is there to facilitate your thinking, not control it. You do not have to have a specific 'problem' to ask for mentoring – the work is focused on developing your professional well being, to support you in getting the best out of your working life.

All mentoring sessions are confidential – the mentor does not have a 'report back' function, either to the Dean of Postgraduate General Practice Education, or anyone else.

As mentoring is seen as an activity which promotes professional development, all mentoring sessions within this South Thames (West) project are eligible for PGEA accreditation.

How do I join the mentoring project?

If you would like to participate in this project, and contribute to our knowledge about the potential contribution of mentoring to general practice, please fill in your name, contact address, and telephone and fax number, and return it to the Mentor Project Co-ordinator, who will then provide you with a mentor. Mentors and mentees are allocated randomly, by the Co-ordinator, who takes into account location and travelling time, and strives to achieve a 'neutral' pairing.

If for any reason you are unhappy with your allocated mentor, then let the Project Co-ordinator know, and she will simply re-allocate.

A freepost envelope is enclosed for your use.

REGIONAL MENTOR PROJECT
MENTEE DETAILS FOR DATABASE

Name:

....
(including Christian name)

Male/Female (Pls circle as appropriate)

Contact address (incl postcode please)

....

....

Contact telephone No. ....

Best time to contact me on the above number: ....

Fax number: ....

Practice address: ....

....

....

Practice phone number: ....

Best time to contact me on the above number: ....

If you are in partnership please indicate how many are in partnership:

....

How many years have you been in partnership? ....

Today's date: ....

Please return this form in the freepost envelope provided to:
Mentor Project Co-ordinator

Appendix 2

MENTOR/MENTEE INTERVIEW RECORDING SHEET

Date: ....

Name (mentor) ....

Name (mentee) ....

CONTENT (including review of earlier key issues):

PERSONAL IMPRESSIONS (How do you think the session went?):

KEY ISSUES EMERGING (including any future objectives):

INTENDED ACTION
By the mentor:

By the mentee:

Date and venue of next meeting:

Appendix 3

SOUTH THAMES (WEST) MENTOR PROJECT

STRICTLY CONFIDENTIAL

**Questionnaire for mentees who have completed
their mentoring sessions**

*Please complete and return this form to the Mentor Project Co-ordinator in the
freepost envelope provided.*

EXPECTATIONS
Can you please say here what your expectations were of mentoring?

Has *anything unexpected* come out of your mentoring experience?

PROCESS
*Can you state briefly what the <u>main themes</u> of your mentoring sessions have
been?*

How professional has the mentoring process been?

OUTCOMES
Can you identify any change in your attitude, behaviour, or circumstances
arising from your mentor experience?

SUGGESTED IMPROVEMENTS
It would be helpful to the Mentor team to have ideas from you about
improving their work.

COMMENTS
Are there any general comments you can add?

Please give your age and indicate whether you are male or female:

....

If in partnership please give details of how many years and the number of

GPs in your partnership ....

THANK YOU
Name: ....

Today's date: ....

Please return in the freepost envelope provided to: (Mentor Project Co-
ordinator).

Appendix 4

POSTGRADUATE MEDICAL EDUCATION FOR GENERAL PRACTICE
South Thames (West)

REGIONAL CRITERIA FOR GP MENTEES, SOUTH THAMES (WEST)

1. Following an initial meeting with his/her mentor, the mentee should complete and return to the Project Co-ordinator the *Initial Interview Form* indicating whether or not he/she wishes to continue for a further three meetings. The mentee is now also given the opportunity of changing to a different mentor.
2. At the end of each of the further three meetings the mentor and mentee will complete together an *Interview Recording Sheet* giving outline details of the session and this will be returned to the Project Co-ordinator.
3. At the conclusion of the third meeting, the mentee and mentor will review the position and decide whether to arrange a further two meetings.
4. At the end of the mentoring sessions the mentee will be required to complete and return an 'Exit' questionnaire giving feedback on their mentoring experience.
5. All information supplied to the Project Co-ordinator in the *Initial Interview Form, Interview Recording Sheet and Exit Questionnaire* is **strictly confidential** and will be seen only by the Co-ordinator and Project Leader.
6. Should mentees wish to rejoin the scheme they can do so by contacting the Project Co-ordinator.
7. The mentor/mentee interviews are accredited for Postgraduate Education Allowance and mentees should claim this by writing to the Dean of Postgraduate General Practice Education stating the time and length of each mentoring session, not including travelling.
8. Mentees should be prepared to travel a reasonable distance (10–15 miles), if necessary, to meet their mentor.
9. Mentoring makes a high demand on the resources from this department. Failure to keep an arranged appointment is, at times, unavoidable, but we do ask you to keep in mind that failed appointments do waste our limited budget.

Dr R.G. Hornung
Dean of Postgraduate General
Practice Education
South Thames (West)

Mrs Rosslynne Freeman
Educational Advisor/
Mentor Project Leader
South Thames (West)

Appendix 5: Database information

The Mentoring Database has been developed to track the movement of mentees through the scheme and provides valuable statistical information on each mentee and mentor. If you are interested in discussing the setting up of your own customized database with our mentoring database consultant please apply to: The Mentoring Project Co-ordinator, Postgraduate Medical Education for General Practice, 2 Stirling House, Stirling Road, Guildford, Surrey GU2 5RF.

Appendix 6: Example of a questionnaire used with mentees to elicit the impact of mentoring on 12 aspects of their professional life

1. Has your effectiveness as a GP

   improved greatly
   improved a little
   not been affected

2. Has your general confidence

   improved greatly
   improved
   remained the same
   deteriorated

3. Has your enthusiasm for your work

   increased greatly
   increased
   remained the same
   lessened

4. Do you think your potential for future professional development

   has been enhanced
   may be enhanced
   is unaffected
   has slowed down

5. Has your ability to cope with stressful situations

   improved greatly
   improved a bit
   not been affected

6. Has your professional knowledge and understanding

   been enhanced
   remained the same
   not been affected

7. Do you think your potential for future personal development has been

   enhanced
   unaffected
   slowed down

8. Have you made any changes to your clinical practice?

   major changes
   minor changes
   none

9. Have you changed any of the services you offer
   patients?

   major changes
   minor changes
   none

10. Have you made any changes in the way you
    manage your practice?

    major changes
    minor changes
    none

11. Have you made any changes in the way you
    work with other members of your team?

    major changes
    some changes
    minor changes
    none

12. Have you made any changes in the way you
    work with other professions?

    major changes
    some changes
    minor changes
    none

Index

Page numbers printed in *italic* refer to tables